# Nanobiotechnology

*Guest Editor*

KEWAL K. JAIN, MD, FFPM

# CLINICS IN LABORATORY MEDICINE

www.labmed.theclinics.com

*Consulting Editor*
ALAN WELLS, MD, DMSc

March 2012 • Volume 32 • Number 1

SAUNDERS an imprint of ELSEVIER, Inc.

**W.B. SAUNDERS COMPANY**
*A Division of Elsevier Inc.*

1600 John F. Kennedy Boulevard • Suite 1800 • Philadelphia, Pennsylvania 19103-2899

http://www.theclinics.com

**CLINICS IN LABORATORY MEDICINE Volume 32, Number 1**
**March 2012 ISSN 0272-2712, ISBN-13: 978-1-4557-3883-0**

Editor: Katie Hartner
Developmental Editor: Donald Mumford

*Reprints.* For copies of 100 or more, of articles in this publication, please contact the Commercial Reprints Department, Elsevier Inc., 360 Park Avenue South, New York, New York 10010-1710. Tel. (212) 633-3813, Fax: (212) 462-1935, E-mail: reprints@elsevier.com.

*Clinics in Laboratory Medicine* (ISSN 0272-2712) is published quarterly by Elsevier Inc., 360 Park Avenue South, New York, NY 10010-1710. Months of issue are March, June, September, and December. Business and Editorial offices: 1600 John F. Kennedy Blvd., Suite 1800, Philadelphia, PA 19103-2899. Periodicals postage paid at NewYork, NY and additional mailing offices. Subscription prices are $240.00 per year (US individuals), $382.00 per year (US institutions), $128.00 (US students), $291.00 per year (Canadian individuals), $483.00 per year (foreign institutions), $176.00 (foreign students). Foreign air speed delivery is included in all *Clinics* subscription prices. All prices are subject to change without notice. POSTMASTER: Send address changes to *Clinics in Laboratory Medicine*, Elsevier Health Sciences Division, Subscription Customer Service, 3251 Riverport Lane, Maryland Heights, MO 63043. **Customer Service: 1-800-654-2452 (US). From outside of the US and Canada, call 1-314-447-8871. Fax: 1-314-447-8029. E-mail: journalscustomerservice-usa@elsevier.com (for print support) or journalsonlinesupport-usa@elsevier.com (for online support).**

*Clinics in Laboratory Medicine* is covered in *EMBASE/Exerpta Medica, MEDLINE/PubMed (Index Medicus), Cinahl, Current Contents/Clinical Medicine, BIOSIS* and *ISI/BIOMED.*

Printed and bound by CPI Group (UK) Ltd, Croydon, CR0 4YY
Transferred to Digital Print 2012

# Contributors

## CONSULTING EDITOR

**ALAN WELLS, MD, DMSc**
Department of Pathology, University of Pittsburgh, Pittsburgh, Pennsylvania

## GUEST EDITOR

**KEWAL K. JAIN, MD, FRACS, FFPM**
Department of Biotechnology, Jain PharmaBiotech, Basel, Switzerland

## AUTHORS

**STEPHEN ALEXANDER, PhD**
Division of Biological Sciences, University of Missouri, Columbia, Missouri

**PEDRO V. BAPTISTA, PhD**
Assistant Professor of Molecular Genetics, Nanotheranostics Group at CIGMH, Departamento de Ciências da Vida, Faculdade de Ciências e Tecnologia, Universidade Nova de Lisboa, Caparica, Portugal

**KIRAN BHATTACHARYYA, BS**
Department of Biological Engineering, University of Missouri, Columbia, Missouri

**GIORGIO FASSINA, PhD**
Xeptagen SpA, Venice, Italy

**ANDREA GALLOTTA, PhD**
Xeptagen SpA, Venice, Italy

**BENJAMIN S. GOLDSCHMIDT, BS**
Department of Biochemistry, University of Missouri, Columbia, Missouri

**MARK HANNINK, PhD**
Department of Biochemistry, Christopher S. Bond Life Sciences Center, University of Missouri, Columbia, Missouri

**KEWAL K. JAIN, MD, FRACS, FFPM**
Department of Biotechnology, Jain PharmaBiotech, Basel, Switzerland

**ALEKSANDER JURKEVIC, PhD**
Molecular Cytology Core, Christopher S. Bond Life Sciences Center, University of Missouri, Columbia, Missouri

**SHIN-ICHIRO NISHIMURA, PhD**
Field of Drug Discovery Research, Faculty of Advanced Life Science, Graduate School of Life Science, Hokkaido University and Medicinal Chemistry Pharmaceuticals LLC, Sapporo, Japan

**ENRICO ORZES, PhD**
Xeptagen SpA, Venice, Italy

**SANDIPAN RAY, MSc, PhD**
Wadhwani Research Center for Biosciences and Bioengineering, Department of
Biosciences and Bioengineering, Indian Institute of Technology Bombay, Powai,
Mumbai, India

**PANGA JAIPAL REDDY, MSc, PhD**
Wadhwani Research Center for Biosciences and Bioengineering, Department of
Biosciences and Bioengineering, Indian Institute of Technology Bombay, Powai,
Mumbai, India.

**SUDIPTA SADHU, BTech, MTech**
Wadhwani Research Center for Biosciences and Bioengineering, Department of
Biosciences and Bioengineering, Indian Institute of Technology Bombay, Powai,
Mumbai, India

**SANJEEVA SRIVASTAVA, PhD**
Wadhwani Research Center for Biosciences and Bioengineering, Department of
Biosciences and Bioengineering, Indian Institute of Technology Bombay, Powai,
Mumbai, India

**JOHN A. VIATOR, PhD**
Departments of Biological Engineering and Dermatology, Christopher S. Bond Life
Sciences Center, University of Missouri, Columbia, Missouri

# Contents

Cancer is the third leading cause of death in developed countries and the second in the United States. Nanotechnology has great potential for early detection, accurate diagnosis, and personalized treatment of cancer. It may provide rapid and sensitive detection of cancer-related molecular alterations, even in a small percentage of cells. Use of gold nanoparticles derivatized with thiol-modified oligonucleotides (Au-nanoprobes) has been gaining momentum as an alternative to more traditional methodologies. Nevertheless, few reports exist on gold nanoparticles for quantitative assessment of gene expression. The application of Au-nanoprobes for assessment of gene expression in cancer is discussed.

Nanobiotechnology has greatly refined the diagnosis of cancer not only by detection of biomarkers and in vitro assays but also by molecular imaging for in vivo diagnosis. The most important advantage of the use of nanoparticles is the opportunity to combine diagnosis with delivery of therapy for cancer. Early detection of cancer, refinement of cancer diagnosis and monitoring of cancer therapy will contribute to the development of personalized therapy of cancer. Rapid advances are taking place in nanobiotechnology, and considerable improvements are expected by its applications to the diagnosis and treatment of cancer.

Many biomarkers have been found overexpressed in neoplastic tissues, and some are used for diagnosis. However, currently used biomarkers have poor sensitivity and specificity mainly because of cancer hetero-geneity. In addition the same types of tumor may produce different biomarkers. Efforts are focusing on the merging of nanotechnologies and biotechnologies to create biochips for detection of several bio-markers at the same time to increase diagnostic accuracy and reduce costs. These devices will allow early detection and identification of many forms of cancer within minutes and directly at the point of care.

Analysis of different biological fluids that contain an archive of information regarding the pathophysiologic conditions of a patient is very useful for biomarker discovery and early disease diagnosis. In recent years, there have been intense efforts to analyze various biological fluids and identify panels of protein markers for different types of cancers. Among the different emerging label-free approaches, surface plasmon resonance (SPR) and SPR imaging are the most promising candidates for diagnostic applications as well as studying biomolecular interactions. This article highlights the key technological advances of SPR-based sensing approaches and their applications in cancer biomarker discovery and inhibitor screening of tumor targets.

Multifunctional phosphorylcholine self-assembled monolayer-coated quantum dots (PCSAM-QDs) displaying glycoconjugates with excellent solubility and long-term stability in aqueous solution without loss of quantum yields were developed. Live animal imaging by PCSAM-QDs displaying various carbohydrates (glyco-PC-QDs) uncovered the evidence of an essential role of the terminal sialic acid residues for achieving prolonged in vivo lifetime and biodistribution of this new class of nanoparticles.

Exploiting the plasmon resonance of gold nanoparticles and the ability to specifically target cancer cell surface proteins, photoacoustic flowmetry may be used to detect nonpigmented circulating tumor cells (CTCs). The authors targeted the EpCAM receptors to attach 50-nm gold nanoparticles to a breast cancer cell line, T47D. After determining the absorption peak and thus the most sensitive laser wavelength, they performed serial dilution trials to show detection of small numbers of breast cancer cells in suspension. This ability may allow an earlier clinical diagnosis and management of metastatic disease for a range of solid tumor types.

## THE CLINICS ARE NOW AVAILABLE ONLINE!

Access your subscription at:
**www.theclinics.com**

# Preface
# Nanobiotechnology-Based Cancer Diagnosis

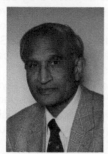

Kewal K. Jain, MD, FRACS, FFPM
*Guest Editor*

Nanobiotechnology has refined molecular diagnosis and extended the limits of detection. This is important for the laboratory diagnosis of cancer as well as for guiding treatment. Several innovations of assays for detection of cancer based on nanobiotechnology are described in this issue of *Clinics in Laboratory Medicine*.

Detection of circulating tumor cells (CTCs) enables early detection of cancer, assessment of prognosis, and monitoring of response to therapy. Methods for detection of CTCs include polymerase chain reaction, microfluidic capture, flow cytometry, and immunomagnetic separation. Bhattacharyya and coworkers describe a technique of CTC detection using antibody-targeted gold nanoparticles and photoacoustic flowmetry. The authors propose that epithelial-mesenchymal transition characteristics of a CTC will be a good predictor of its ability to metastasize and it is worthwhile to develop assays for determining this.

Biomarkers play an important role in the detection of cancer but many of the currently available biomarkers lack specificity and sensitivity. Gallotta and colleagues have shown how nanobiotechnologies combined with biochips can be used for the simultaneous detection of several cancer biomarkers with increased sensitivity and low cost. Assays have been developed for characterizing a particular DNA sequence in cancer. Baptista describes the application of gold nanoparticles for the quantitative assessment of posttranscriptional gene expression in cancer, which also plays an important role in the development of cancer. The use of nanoparticles for quantitative measurement of RNA will refine further cancer diagnosis.

Most of the detection systems for cancer biomarkers use labeling procedures, which are time-consuming and limit the number and types of analytes that can be studied simultaneously. Reddy and colleagues have presented surface plasmon resonance (SPR)-based nanosensors as a label-free approach for high-throughput screening of specific biomarkers of various cancers. The authors have pointed out limitations of the

Clin Lab Med 32 (2012) ix–x
doi:10.1016/j.cll.2012.01.002
0272-2712/12/$ – see front matter © 2012 Elsevier Inc. All rights reserved.

application of SPR-based immunoassay of SPR in routine clinical diagnostics and the efforts that are being made to overcome these, including the use of nanoparticles.

Nanoparticle-based in vivo molecular imaging for the detection of cancer and the guidance of treatment is making rapid progress. Materials used to synthesize nanoparticles include natural proteins, glycans, polymers, dendrimers, fullerenes, and metals. Glycans are promising signal molecules for controlled targeted drug delivery of biopharmaceuticals. Nishimura and coworkers describe a method for the preparation of multifunctional QDs (PCSAM-QDs) displaying glycoconjugates with excellent solubility in aqueous solution without loss of quantum yields. Passage of PCSAM-QDs in live animals can be followed using versatile near-infrared fluorescence photometry. This novel technology has potential applications in oncology.

As pointed out in some of the articles in this issue, nanoparticle-based assays for cancer will facilitate the development of personalized oncology. Jain has reviewed the role of nanotechnology in the detection of cancer biomarkers, early diagnosis of cancer, in vivo cancer imaging, and the combination of diagnosis with therapeutics, which are important components of personalized therapy of cancer.

Kewal K. Jain, MD, FRACS, FFPM
Department of Biotechnology
Jain PharmaBiotech
Blaesiring 7
Basel 4057, Switzerland

E-mail address:
jain@pharmabiotech.ch

# RNA Quantification with Gold Nanoprobes for Cancer Diagnostics

Pedro V. Baptista, PhD*

KEYWORDS

- Gold nanoparticles
- RNA quantification
- Cancer
- Nanodiagnostics
- Molecular diagnostics
- RNA

Cancer is the third leading cause of death after heart disease and stroke in developed countries and the second leading cause of death after heart disease in the United States.[1] It is projected that the number of new cases of all cancers worldwide will be 12.3 million in 2010 and 15.4 million in 2020.[2] More than 1.5 million new cancer cases and about one-half million deaths from cancer are projected to occur in 2010 in the United States alone.[3] Nanotechnology, an interdisciplinary research field involving chemistry, engineering, biology, and medicine, has great potential for early detection, accurate diagnosis, and personalized treatment of cancer.[4,5] Molecular nanodiagnostics applied to cancer may provide rapid and sensitive detection of cancer-related molecular alterations, which would enable early detection even when those alterations occur only in a small percentage of cells. The use of gold nanoparticles derivatized with thiol-modified oligonucleotides (Au-nanoprobes) for the detection of specific nucleic acid targets has been gaining momentum as an alternative to more traditional methodologies. Nevertheless, few reports exist on application of gold nanoparticles for quantitative assessment of gene expression. Here, the application of Au-nanoprobes for gene expression in cancer is discussed.

## BACKGROUND
### Molecular Aspects in Cancer Diagnostics

Cancer is a complex group of diseases resulting from the interaction between the genome and the environment to which that same genome is exposed. Many of the

This work was supported by Fundação para a Ciência e Tecnologia/Ministério apra a Ciência e Tecnologia e Ensino Superior Grant to Centro de Investigação em Genética Molecular Humana. The author has nothing to disclose.

Nanotheranostics Group at CIGMH, Departamento de Ciências da Vida, Faculdade de Ciências e Tecnologia, Universidade Nova de Lisboa, Caparica, Portugal

* Corresponding author. Nanothernostics Group at CIGMH, Departamento de Ciências da Vida, Faculdade de Ciências e Tecnologia, Universidade Nova de Lisboa, Campus de Caparica, 2829-516 Caparica, Portugal.
E-mail address: pmvb@fct.unl.pt

Clin Lab Med 32 (2012) 1–13
doi:10.1016/j.cll.2011.09.001
0272-2712/12/$ – see front matter © 2012 Elsevier Inc. All rights reserved.

molecular alterations observed in cancer originate at the DNA sequence level and can be classified as (a) germline (inherited and shared by all cells in the body) or (b) somatic (occurring during mitosis and confined to a specific cell population, tissue, and/or organ).[6–10] Several other molecular events may increase the risk of cancer development and progression, such as epigenetic mechanisms (eg, DNA methylation, histone modification, and micro RNA [miRNA] regulation).[11,12] These events are not genetic alterations because they do not alter the initial DNA sequence but rather modulate the way that same sequence might be expressed into RNA and further into protein. For example, germline mutations in the TP53 and BRCA1 genes are associated with a high lifetime risk of breast and other cancers.[13,14] TP53 is a tumor suppressor gene whose protein is produced in response to DNA damage, resulting in cell cycle arrest in G1 and induction of pathways leading to DNA repair or apoptosis. Mutation in the TP53 gene leading to decreased p53 activity may result in cells with DNA damage to override cell cycle arrest, thus continuing to replicate with damaged DNA. In the case of BRCA1, the majority of confirmed mutations generate truncated proteins that are likely to have severely reduced activity.

Chromosome instability describes an increased rate of chromosome missegregation in mitosis leading to an aberrant chromosomal state such as changes in ploidy, gain or loss of whole chromosomes (aneuploidy), or chromosomal rearrangements, all of which are hallmarks of cancers. Such an example is chronic myeloid leukemia (CML), a clonal neoplastic disease of the hematopoietic stem cell, whose hallmark molecular event is the genetic t(9;22)(q34;q11) translocation known as the Philadelphia chromosome.[15,16] This translocation—*ABL* gene (chromosome 9) and *BCR* gene (chromosome 22)—originates a *BCR-ABL* fusion gene, leading to the expression of a chimeric BCR-ABL protein with tyrosine-kinase activity.[17–19]

Genetic variations or polymorphisms existing in the human genome can also confer genetic susceptibility to cancer. The Human Genome Project made huge amounts of data available, and high numbers of genetic polymorphisms have been discovered,[20] creating unprecedented opportunities to study and understand the consequences of genetic variations. One of the great challenges of modern molecular biology is integration of genetic information into procedures that can be implemented in rapid, cost-effective, and reliable methods to genotype, phenotype, and identify gene function. There are several types of polymorphisms in the human genome (eg, insertions and/or deletions of one or more bases, duplications), but single nucleotide polymorphisms (SNPs) are the more frequent (~68%).[21,22] Several million SNPs have been reported in various databases and associated with susceptibility to disease.[23–25] These databases include Celera Human Ref SNP,[26] National Center for Biotechnology Information dbSNP,[27] Human Genome Variation Database-HGVbase,[28] The Human Gene Mutation Database-HGMD,[29] and HapMap Project.[30] SNPs are widespread in the human genome: (i) located in a coding region may modify the activity of a protein (nonsynonymous SNP/missense SNP), (ii) located in the boundary exon/intron could modify the splicing process, (iii) other intronic SNPs and synonymous SNPs (base changes in the coding region that do not cause an amino acid change) could also change messenger RNA (mRNA) stability with potential implications for gene expression, (iv) located in the promoter region or intragenic regions may lead to enhancement and/silencing mechanisms.[31] Individual genetic variability as a consequence of SNPs has been associated with individual susceptibility to multifactorial diseases such as cancer and provides for the study of effective molecular biomarkers for cancer and for the development of targeted molecular screening techniques.

Molecular diagnostics in cancer require highly paralleled and miniaturized assays capable of incorporating the vast information made available by the genome sequencing and genome analysis projects. Thus far, most diagnostic methods focus on detection of the response mechanisms of disease (eg, antibody produced by the organism in response to cellular transformation). Such methods are slow and lack efficiency because they involve recognizing a disease based on the patient developing the disease first. Alternatively, technologies based on nucleic acid characterization aim at detecting the disease/condition, and/or even the probability of developing a specific condition before the individual shows the symptoms. Historically, detection of DNA has been carried out using either radioactive or organic fluorophore labeling of the probe molecule, such as DNA chips for highly parallelized throughput.[32,33] Especially for the highly integrated DNA chips, fluorescence labeling for nucleic acid characterization became the method of choice because of the high sensitivity and ease of use. Although fluorescence detection is widely used, it also exhibits some problems, for example low stability of the dyes, influence of the physicochemical environment on signal intensity, and expensive setup for filtering the exciting and emitting light used for detection. Nevertheless, recent advances in dissecting the somatic mutational profile of cancer genomes have been driven by high-throughput or next-generation sequencing technologies based on fluorescence signals.[34,35] Many large-scale targeted resequencing studies of collections of cancer-relevant candidate genes, gene families, or all the RefSeq (Reference Sequence) Database genes had been previously characterized in individual, more focused studies aimed at providing insights into cancer genomics.[36,37]

## The Case for RNA-Based Assays

Despite the focus on the critical role of DNA in cancer onset and development and consequent development of assays for characterizing a particular DNA sequence, there has been accumulating evidence supporting the role of posttranscriptional gene regulation in the development of cancer.[38] In fact, cancer development and mechanisms of disease progression have been associated with perturbations of ordinary RNA processing events such as defects in alternative premessenger RNA splicing, alternative splicing of tumor suppressors and oncogenes, differential mRNA localization, and expression in regulation of cell death together with ever increasing involvement of epigenetic factors (eg, miRNA silencing and activation; gene methylation).[39-45] Therefore microarrays have been at the forefront of gene expression studies in cancer. Similarly, RNA-Seq has recently been used to assess expression levels of both coding and noncoding transcripts where their abundance is proportional to the number of sequence reads and for identifying genes associated with cancer development.[46,47] Circulating extracellular mRNA and miRNA are growingly considered the next generation of cancer biomarkers.[48-50]

One point that should be kept in mind is that the ability to study and compare the expression of mRNA populations from different samples has become possible by the application of reverse transcription (RT), usually combined with polymerase chain reaction (PCR).[51] This way, with the exception of those technologies that rely on the hybridization of a labeled probe directly to RNA (eg, fluorescence in situ hybridization, Northern blot), all available platforms require a prior step of retrotranscription in order to convert the mRNA into complementary DNA (cDNA) that is then characterized (**Fig. 1**). This step is of the utmost relevance when assessing and developing a technology for RNA detection, characterization, and/or quantification, because the enzymatic step mediated by reverse transcriptase is definitely not free of error and of stochastic bias that may hamper effective evaluation of the molecular aspects involved.

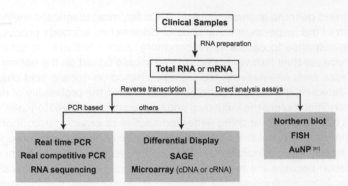

Fig. 1. Overview of RNA quantification. The steps required to attain total RNA are not referred. It should be noted that in order to attain total RNA, often smaller RNA fragments (eg, miRNAs) may be lost and/or underrepresented in final sample to be assayed. It is well-known that retrotranscription shows some pitfalls (eg, stochastic enzymatic action, inhibition by common reagents and ionic conditions, some RNAs contain secondary structures that hamper reverse transcriptase action), and these limitations will cause efficiency problems and lack of consistency. PCR analysis assays refers to assays that require/are based upon the use of enzymatic amplification of cDNA prior to the detection step.

## NANODIAGNOSTICS FOR CANCER

The National Cancer Institute envisions that over the next years nanotechnology will result in significant advances in early detection, molecular imaging, targeted and multifunctional therapeutics, and prevention and control of cancer.[52] Nanodiagnostics is a burgeoning field of research and development providing for more and improved techniques toward clinical diagnostics with increased sensitivity at lower costs.[5,53–56] Recent progress in nanotechnology and DNA-nanoparticle conjugate systems (eg, quantum dots and noble metal nanoparticles) have been shown to be extremely powerful tools for the development of molecular assays.[57–67] Applications of nanotechnology in molecular diagnostics are likely to extend the limits of contemporary molecular diagnostic techniques. Nanotechnology implemented within current diagnostic equipment has the potential of analyzing entire genomes in minutes instead of hours. Working at the nanoscale also decreases the cost associated with genetic tests and the amount of sample needed. Based on which DNA sequences are deviated from the normal (SNPs and mutations), doctors may be able to determine an individual's predisposition to cancer or any other specific disease with genetic input. The field of nanodiagnostics also sees a trend toward hand-held devices that are easy to use and marketable to be used at point of care by doctors and other health care professionals. The possibility of personalized medicine is conveyed by the conjugation of properties associated with nanoparticles such as quantum dots and/or gold nanoparticles (AuNPs) that can be used to refine biomarkers for molecular diagnostics and as vectors for targeted drug delivery and could enable early detection of cancer and more effective and less toxic treatment, increasing the chances of cure. New devices include nanovectors for the targeted delivery of anticancer drugs and imaging contrast agents.[58,68]

Until now, these DNA-nanoparticle conjugates have been used extensively as a biomolecular label for specific oligonucleotide probes capable of discriminating complementary target sequences.[60] Many of these nanotechnology-based systems have been applied to the characterization of sequences of genes associated with cancer. However, most of these proposed platforms have yet to be applied to biological and/or clinical samples in order to prove their effective use as diagnostic tools (see, for example, Baptista and colleagues' **Table 1**[60]). Nevertheless, some have demonstrated their capability of detecting mutations in genes responsible for cancer development. For example, Li and colleagues[69] used AuNPs to enhance the detection capability of a point mutation in the BRCA1 gene at a concentration of 1pM, a key gene involved in familiar breast and ovarian cancer. Further sensitivity without loss of selectivity was achieved by use of silver nanoparticles for chemiluminescent SNP detection on fragments of the human p53 gene at concentrations as low as 5fM.[70]

Because of their remarkable properties, noble metal nanoparticles have been particularly a focus when developing biomolecular sensing platforms.[60] Metal nanoparticles, usually constituted by clustered metal atoms (3 to $10^7$ atoms) protected by a capping agent, exhibit remarkable properties, such as highly tunable spectral behavior and high surface/volume ratios. Noteworthy are the amazing optical properties—intense color and high scattering of light—due to the localized surface plasmon resonance (LSPR).[71,72] This concept may be explained as the collective oscillations of free electrons at a metal-dielectric interface, when the frequency of incident light coincides with the frequency of electron oscillation, resulting in a surface plasmon resonance (SPR). These oscillations originate the intense colors and/or very intense scattering of the colloidal dispersions of nanoparticles and are strongly influenced by the nanoparticles' size, dispersion, shape, and composition.[73–79] Gold nanoparticles sized between 2 and 40 nm exhibit a typical LSPR band centered at around 520 nm that can be easily synthesized via reduction of a gold salt,[74] yielding stable colloidal solutions. These AuNPs can be used directly in colorimetric DNA detection schemes capable of discriminating SNPs within the target sequence.[80–83] These AuNPs can also be directly functionalized with thiol-modified oligonucleotides,[84] resulting in what is known as gold-nanoprobes (Au-nanoprobes) that can be used in a multitude of detection strategies for recognition of specific nucleic acid sequences.[60,85–87]

## GOLD NANOPARTICLES FOR RNA DETECTION

Despite the high number of detection schemes presented in the literature for DNA detection and characterization, few reports can be found for detection and/or quantification of RNA. It should, however, be mentioned that once a retrotranscription step is introduced to create cDNA, most of the proposed DNA-based nanodiagnostics systems can be used for indirectly assessing and quantifying expression of a given gene or sequence. However, for small RNAs such as miRNAs and short mRNA transcripts, this prior step may be very limiting, and reliable results can only be attained via direct questioning of the RNA molecule. Also, expression analysis typically requires target labeling, usually achieved by RT of the RNA sample to incorporate labeled nucleotides into the growing cDNA strand. As in every retrotranscription-based method, in cases of limiting starting material, production of cDNA may not yield enough target molecules for the downstream detection procedure.

The first AuNP-based approach for RNA detection was reported by Cao and colleagues[88] in 2002, using oligonucleotides probes labeled with AuNPs and Raman-active dyes for multiplexed detection of oligonucleotide targets. These probes consist of 13 nm AuNPs functionalized with Raman dye–labeled oligonucleotides. The Raman spectroscopic fingerprint, which can be designed through choice of Raman label, can be identified after silver enhancing by scanning Raman spectroscopy. This approach was developed for a DNA detection scheme and then applied for discriminating and quantifying two synthetic RNA oligonucleotides differing by a single base pair; in other words, an SNP. Despite this fingerprinting method offering potentially greater flexibility and higher multiplexing capabilities than conventional fluorescence-based detection approaches, its application directly to biological RNA samples has not been reported.

Another method using AuNPs for quantitative analysis of RNA was presented by Huber and colleagues[89] and used an oligo-$dT_{20}$–modified gold nanoparticle probe for detection of microarray-bound RNA molecules by targeting the poly-A tail. Further enhancement of the hybridization is achieved via autometallography, and subsequent measurement of nanoparticle-mediated light scattering. This high sensitivity afforded by the Au-nanoprobes allows differential gene expression from as little as 0.5 mg unamplified total human RNA in a 2 h hybridization without the need for elaborate sample labeling steps. To demonstrate the dynamic performance of the method, 13 human genes representing high-, medium-, low-, and nonexpressed transcripts were used as a model system to test the concept of hybridizing total human RNA. Because hybridization recognizes the poly-A tail present in most eukaryotic transcripts, the Au-nanoprobe provide for multiparallel expression analysis that accounts for semi-quantitative measurements. The method demonstrated lack of a 3′ end bias, suggesting that splice variants can be detected and quantified. Despite all the advantages, this approach does not allow for recognition and targeting of miRNAs.

Detection of miRNA expression has since been reported by Liang and colleagues[90] using an oligonucleotide microarray based on labeling RNA with quantum dot and Au-nanoprobe. In this miRNA profiling microarray, miRNAs were directly labeled at the 3′ end with biotin and hybridized to complementary DNA oligonucleotide probes immobilized on glass slides and subsequently detected by measuring fluorescence of quantum dots labeled with streptavidin that bind to miRNAs through streptavidin-biotin interaction. The presented results were consistent with the Northern blot result. Analysis of a model microarray indicated that the detection limit for miRNA was 0.4 fmol and the detection dynamic range spanned about 2 orders of magnitude, from 0.16 to 20 nM. Nevertheless, this system requires direct labeling of the target molecules (miRNAs), which can considerably hamper detection because of differential efficiencies in labeling of underrepresented molecules. It should also be mentioned that the proposed system has not been applied to human miRNAs nor to cancer-related miRNAs in circulation; in other words, no data are available on suitability for cancer biomarkers detection application.

## GOLD NANOPARTICLES FOR RNA QUANTIFICATION—APPLICATION TO CANCER DIAGNOSTICS

In 2005, Baptista and colleagues[91] reported on the specific detection of mRNA expression using gold nanoparticles functionalized with thiol–single-stranded DNA (ssDNA). The detection scheme is based on a noncrosslinking hybridization method, in which aggregation of the Au-nanoprobes is induced by an increasing salt concentration. The method consists of visual and/or spectrophotometric comparison of solutions before and after salt-induced Au-nanoprobe aggregation—the presence of complementary target prevents aggregation, and the solution remains red; non-complementary/mismatched targets do not prevent Au-nanoprobe aggregation resulting in a visible change of color from red to blue. This Au-nanoprobe method was used to detect eukaryotic gene expression (RNA) without the need for retrotranscription or PCR amplification steps directly from as little as 0.3 $\mu$g of unamplified total RNA, avoiding the RNA to cDNA conversion step normally used by other methods. The robustness and effectiveness of the proposed noncrosslinking method has been further demonstrated by application of the detection scheme to pathogens and SNP detection[92–94] without the need for cumbersome laboratory equipment and with the possibility of incorporation into a portable detection platform.[95]

Based on this approach, the same group reported on the use of this Au-nanoprobe system for the specific detection and quantification of the BCR-ABL transcript, which is responsible for CML (see above - BACKGROUND: Molecular aspects in cancer diagnostics section).[96] The Au-nanoprobe–based approach was used for the molecular recognition and quantification of *BCR-ABL* b3a2 (e14a2) fusion for the early diagnosis of CML using total human RNA as target without RT and/or amplification. The Au-nanoprobe sequences were specifically designed to target the normal gene transcripts, BCR and ABL, and the fusion product by overlapping the fusion region of the transcript. Detection capability was proven by using total RNA extracted from K562 erythroleukemic cells (*BCR-ABL*–positive cell line derived from CML patients in blast crisis) and HL-60 cell line, a human leukemic promyelocytic cell line (*BCR-ABL*– negative). It should be noted that in reality, patients may only harbor one copy of the fusion gene, and the remaining copies of normal *ABL* and *BCR* should be still functional, thus expressing the normal mRNA sequence. Therefore, two oligonucleotides, each harboring the normal sequence of the *BCR* and *ABL* genes, respectively, were used to evaluate the strategy's capability to discriminate from similar sequences. This Au-nanoprobe strategy allowed for detection of less than 100 fmol/$\mu$l of a specific RNA target, with the possibility of discriminating between a positive and negative from as little as 10 ng/$\mu$l of total RNA. This strategy was also successfully used to detect the fusion transcript directly from blood of CML patients (João Conde, personal communication, February 2010). Furthermore, the presented methodology was the first report on quantification of human mRNA directly from total RNA without RT or amplification targeting a clear biomarker for cancer diagnostics. Quantification was made possible by assessing the ratio of nonaggregated (SPR peak at 520 nm) and aggregated (SPR peak at 650 nm) of AU-nanoprobe in solution, and using a calibration curve.

The same investigators later demonstrated the use of alloy metal nanoparticles for multicolor cancer diagnostics.[97] Nanoparticles with variable silver and gold compositions in an alloy format were synthesized and functionalized with thiol-modified ssDNA (nanoprobes).[98] These alloys combine the remarkable optical properties of Ag nanoparticles (high extinction coefficient) with the ease of functionalization via a thiol bond provided by the gold. These nanoprobes were then used for the simultaneous specific identification of several mRNA targets involved in cancer development—one-pot multicolor detection of cancer expression. The different metal composition in the alloy yields different"colors" that can be used as tags for identification of a given target. Following the same noncrosslinking hybridization procedure previously described for gold nanoprobes, these multicolor nanoprobes were used for the molecular recognition of several different targets including different variants of gene products involved in CML (eg, BCR, ABL, BCR-ABL fusion product). Based on the spectral signature of mixtures before and after induced aggregation of metal nanoparticles, the correct identification could be made (**Fig. 2**). Further application to differentially quantify expression of each locus in relation to another was also demonstrated using the spectral information as described previously for the Au-nanoprobes.

## SUMMARY

Every day new potential biomarkers for cancer diagnostics are scrutinized by researchers trying to understand the molecular and cellular mechanisms underlying cancer onset and development. Current technologies for nucleic acid characterization

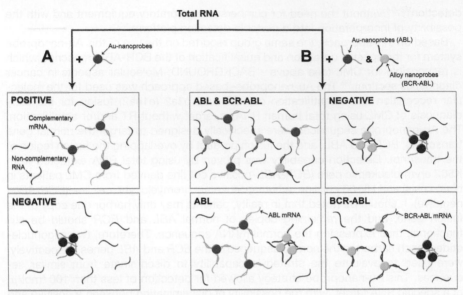

**Fig. 2.** Au-nanoprobe for RNA quantification in cancer. The steps involved in detection of specific RNA (BCR-ABL gene fusion transcript) used as cancer biomarker for CML using total RNA as starting material. Color represents the actual color of the nanoprobe solution. ABL: ABL gene; BCR-ABL: BCR-ABL fusion transcript; NEGATIVE: no complementary target to nanoprobe. (*A*) Detection strategy using Au-nanoprobes alone showing that, upon salt-induced aggregation of the Au-nanoprobes, the presence of the complementary transcript stabilizes the nanoparticles and the solution remains red. The level of nonaggregated/aggregated Au-nanoprobes is used to assess amount of target mRNA in solution. (*B*) One-pot dual-color detection scheme using two sets of nanoprobes, one using Au-nanoparticles and the other using gold: silver alloy nanoparticles. Upon induction of aggregation via salt addition, differential aggregation profiles are noted depending on presence/absence of complementary RNA. Quantification can be made via measuring the ratio of nonaggregated/aggregated nanoprobes.

have been focused on increasing the throughput capability without compromising sensitivity.

Nevertheless, if personalized medicine is to be pursued toward better diagnostics and treatment, a more focused approach capable of being used at the point of need is required. It is here that medium-throughput highly sensitive techniques capable of incorporating up-to-date information provided for the massive efforts into the molecular aspects of cancer development into easy-to-use, simple, and affordable platforms for diagnostics. Nanotechnology-based systems could provide the tools for this unique yet vast niche, offering the technical strategies for personalized medicine in cancer. Nanoparticle-based colorimetric assays for diagnostics has been a subject of intensive research, in which the changes in the local index of refraction upon adsorption of the target molecule to the metal surface can be used to detect DNA or proteins. Because of the intense LSPR in the visible spectrum yielding extremely bright colors, gold nanoparticle colloids have been widely used in molecular diagnostics. In fact, AuNPs functionalized with ssDNA capable of specifically hybridizing to a complementary target for the detection of specific nucleic acid sequences in biological samples have been extensively used. Because of their properties, AuNPs are suitable to be used in protocols for identification of mutation detection and SNPs discrimination associated with disease. Most of the current platforms are focused on increasing sensitivity and/or throughput ratios, but they still rely on highly intensive and specialized technical input with previous sample treatment.

The majority of methods presented thus far constitute interesting concepts in need of validation in real human samples. Also, most applications of nanoparticle-based approaches have been demonstrated in simpler conditions, such as with synthetic oligonucleotides as targets and viruses, which, although relevant for conceptualization are still far away from the severe strains of clinical diagnostics strategies. Although very few approaches have been applied for RNA quantification in real biological samples, current retrotranscription steps can be introduced so as to allow widespread application of nanotechnology-based DNA detection schemes to the cDNA image originated from the sample. This way, a plethora of new RNA characterization platforms can soon make their way into the clinical setting, adding a range of dynamic weapons in cancer diagnostics.

## ACKNOWLEDGMENTS

The author acknowledges FCT/MCTES (Portugal)—CIGMH for financial support, and G. Doria for help with the artwork and valuable discussion.

## REFERENCES

1. Centers for Disease Control and Prevention. Available at: http://www.cdc.gov. Accessed August 10, 2011.
2. Parkin DM. Global cancer statistics in the year 2000. Lancet Oncol 2001;2:533–43.
3. Jemal A, Siegel R, Xu J, et al. Cancer statistics, 2010. CA Cancer J Clin 2010;60: 277–300.
4. Jain KK. Advances in the field of nanooncology. BMC Medicine 2010;8:83.
5. Choi YE, Kwak JW, Park JW. Nanotechnology for early cancer detection. Sensors 2010;10:428–55.
6. Balmain A, Gray J, Ponder B. The genetics and genomics of cancer. Nat Genet 2003;33(Suppl):238–44.
7. Hanahan D, Weinberg RA. The hallmarks of cancer. Cell 2000;100:57–70.
8. Stratton MR, Campbell PJ, Futreal PA. The cancer genome. Nature 2009;458: 719–24.
9. Bell DW. Our changing view of the genomic landscape of cancer. J Pathol 2010;220: 231–43.
10. Harris TJ, McCormick F. The molecular pathology of cancer. Nat Rev Clin Oncol 2010;7:251–65.
11. Sharma S, Kelly TK, Jones PA. Epigenetics in cancer. Carcinogenesis 2010;31: 27–36.
12. Iacobuzio-Donahue CA. Epigenetic changes in cancer. Annu Rev Pathol 2009;4: 229–49.
13. Irminger-Finger I, Jefford CE. Is there more to BARD1 than BRCA1? Nat Rev Cancer 2006;6:382–91.
14. Lewis PD, Parry JM. In silico p53 mutation hotspots in lung cancer. Carcinogenesis 2004;25:1099–107.
15. Hehlmann R, Hochhaus A, Baccarani M. Chronic myeloid leukaemia. Lancet 2007; 370:342–50.
16. Shet AS, Jahagirdar BN, Verfaillie CM. Chronic myelogenous leukemia: mechanisms underlying disease progression. Leukemia 2002;16:1402–11.

17. Ren R. Mechanisms of BCR-ABL in the pathogenesis of chronic myelogenous leukaemia. Nat Rev Cancer 2005;5:172–83.
18. Wong S, Witte ON. The BCR-ABL story: bench to bedside and back. Annu Rev Immunol 2004;22:247–306.
19. Melo J. Inviting leukemic cells to waltz with the devil. Nat Med 2001;7:156–57.
20. Goodstadt L, Ponting CP. Sequence variation and disease in the wake of the draft human genome. Hum Mol Genet 2001;10:2209–14.
21. Weber JL, David D, Heil J, et al. Human diallelic insertion/deletion polymorphisms. Am J Hum Genet 2002;71:854–62.
22. den Dunnen JT, Antonarakis SE. Nomenclature for the description of human sequence variations. Hum Genet 2001;109:121–4.
23. Human mutation databases. UK HGMP Resource Center. Available at: http://www.biologie.uni-hamburg.de/b-online/library/genomeweb/GenomeWeb/human-gen-db-mutation.html. Accessed August 10, 2011.
24. Tabor HK, Risch NJ, Myers RM. Candidate-gene approaches for studying complex genetic traits: practical considerations. Nat Rev Genet 2002;3:391–97.
25. Wheeler DL, Church DM, Federhen S, et al. Database resources of the National Center for Biotechnology. Nucleic Acids Res 2003;31:28–33.
26. Celera. Available at: http://www.celera.com. Accessed August 10, 2011.
27. dbSNP Short genetic variations. National Center for Biotechnology Information. Available at: http://www.ncbi.nlm.nih.gov/SNP/index.html. Accessed August 10, 2011.
28. GWAS Central. A genotype-phenotype association database. Available at: http://www.gwascentral.org. Accessed August 10, 2011.
29. The human gene mutation database. Available at: http://www.hgmd.org. Accessed August 10, 2011.
30. International HapMap Project. Available at: http://snp.cshl.org. Accessed August 10, 2011.
31. Tan IB, Ngeow J, Tan P. Role of polymorphisms in cancer susceptibility. eLS; 2010.
32. Maskos U, Southern EM. Oligonucleotide hybridizations on glass supports: a novel linker for oligonucleotide synthesis and hybridization properties of oligonucleotides synthesised in situ. Nucleic Acids Res 1992;20:1679–84.
33. Schena M, Shalon D, Davis RW, et al. Quantitative monitoring of gene expression patterns with a complementary DNA microarray. Science 1995;270:467–70.
34. Mardis ER. Next-generation DNA sequencing methods. Annu Rev Genomics Hum Genet 2008;9:387–402.
35. Metzker ML. Sequencing technologies - the next generation. Nat Rev Genet 2010;11:31–46.
36. Chee-Seng K, En Yun L, Yudi P, et al. Next generation sequencing technologies and their applications. eLS; 2010.
37. Su Z, Ning B, Fang H, et al. Next-generation sequencing and its applications in molecular diagnostics. Expert Rev Mol Diagn 2011;11:333–43.
38. Copeland NG, Jenkins NA. Deciphering the genetic landscape of cancer – from genes to pathways. Trends Genet 2009;25:455–62.
39. van Kouwenhove M, Kedde M, Agami R. MicroRNA regulation by RNA-binding proteins and its implications for cancer. Nat Rev Cancer 2011;11:644–56.
40. Ballestar E. An introduction to epigenetics. Adv Exp Med Biol 2011;711:1–11.
41. Croce CM. miRNAs in the spotlight: understanding cancer gene dependency. Nat Med 2011;17:935–6.
42. Hager GL, McNally JG, Misteli T. Transcription dynamics. Mol Cell 2009;35:741–53.

43. David CJ, Manley JL. Alternative pre-mRNA splicing regulation in cancer: pathways and programs unhinged. Genes Dev 2010;24:2343–64.
44. Inui M, Martello G, Piccolo S. MicroRNA control of signal transduction. Nat Rev Mol Cell Biol 2010;11:252–63.
45. Dykxhoorn DM. MicroRNAs and metastasis: little RNAs go a long way. Cancer Res 2010;70:6401–6.
46. Hawkins RD, Hon GC, Ren B. Next-generation genomics: an integrative approach. Nat Rev Genet 2010;11:476–86.
47. Wang Z, Gerstein M, Snyder M. RNA-Seq: a revolutionary tool for transcriptomics. Nat Rev Genet 2009;10:57–63.
48. Schwarzenbach H, Hoon DS, Pantel K. Cell-free nucleic acids as biomarkers in cancer patients. Nat Rev Cancer 2011;11:426–37.
49. Munker R, Calin GA. MicroRNA profiling in cancer. Clin Sci (Lond) 2011;121:141–58.
50. Mendrick DL. Transcriptional profiling to identify biomarkers of disease and drug response. Pharmacogenomics 2011;12:235–49.
51. Woodgate L, Mills K. Reverse Transcription and PCR. eLS; 2003.
52. National Cancer Institute. NCI Alliance for Nanotechnology in Cancer. Available at: http://nano.cancer.gov/. Accessed August 10, 2011.
53. Hede S, Huilgol N. "Nano": the new nemesis of cancer. J Cancer Res Ther 2006;2: 186–95.
54. Baptista P. Cancer nanotechnology - prospects for cancer diagnostics and therapy. Curr Cancer Ther Rev 2009;5:80–8.
55. Selvan ST, Tan TT, Yi DK, et al. Functional and multifunctional nanoparticles for bioimaging and biosensing. Langmuir 2010;26:11631–41.
56. Jain KK. Role of nanobiotechnology in developing personalized medicine for cancer. Technol Cancer Res Treat 2005;4:645–50.
57. Condon A. Designed DNA molecules: principles and applications of molecular nanotechnology. Nat Rev Genet 2006;7:565–75.
58. Ferrari M. Cancer nanotechnology: opportunities and challenges. Nat Rev Cancer 2005;5:161–71.
59. Liu CH, Li ZP, Du BA, et al. Silver nanoparticle-based ultrasensitive chemiluminescent detection of DNA hybridization and single-nucleotide polymorphisms. Anal Chem 2006;78:3738–44.
60. Baptista P, Pereira E, Eaton P, et al. Gold nanoparticles for the development of clinical diagnosis methods. Anal Bioanal Chem 2008;391:943–50.
61. Huang X, Jain PK, El-Sayed IH, et al. Gold nanoparticles: interesting optical properties and recent applications in cancer diagnostics and therapy. Nanomedicine (Lond) 2007;2:681–93.
62. Vo-Dinh T, Wang H, Scaffidi J. Plasmonic nanoprobes for SERS biosensing and bioimaging. J Biophotonics 2010;3:89–102.
63. Aslan K, Huang J, Wilson GM, et al. Metal-enhanced fluorescence-based RNA sensing. J Am Chem Soc 2006;128:4206–7.
64. Sun L, Irudayaraj J. PCR-free quantification of multiple splice variants in a cancer gene by surface-enhanced Raman spectroscopy. J Phys Chem B 2009;113:14021–5.
65. Noor M, Goyal S, Christensen S, et al. Electrical detection of single-base DNA mutation using functionalized nanoparticles. Appl Phys Let 2009;95:073703.
66. Han G, Xing Z, Dong Y, et al. One-step homogeneous DNA assay with single-nanoparticle detection. Angew Chem Int Ed Engl 2011;50:3462–5.
67. Qiu F, Gu K, Yang B, et al. DNA assay based on monolayer-barcoded nanoparticles for mass spectrometry in combination with magnetic microprobes. Talanta 2011;85: 1698–702.

68. Pissuwan D, Valenzuela SM, Cortie MB. Therapeutic possibilities of plasmonically heated gold nanoparticles. Trends Biotechnol 2006;24:62–7.
69. Li Y, Wark AW, Lee HJ, et al. Single-nucleotide polymorphism genotyping by nano-particle-enhanced surface plasmon resonance imaging measurements of surface ligation reactions. Anal Chem 2006;78:3158–64.
70. Yao X, Li X, Toledo F, et al. Sub-attomole oligonucleotide and p53 cDNA determina-tions via a high-resolution surface plasmon resonance combined with oligonucle-otide-capped gold nanoparticle signal amplification. Anal Biochem 2006;354:220–8.
71. Moores A, Goettmann F. The plasmon band in noble metal nanoparticles: an intro-duction to theory and applications. New J Chem 2006;30:1121–32.
72. Schasfoort RB, Schuck P. Future trends in SPR technology. In: Schasfoort RB, Tudos AJ, editors. Handbook of surface plasmon resonance. Cambridge (UK): RSC; 2008. p. 354–94.
73. Guler U, Turan R. Effect of particle properties and light polarization on the plasmonic resonances in metallic nanoparticles. Opt Express 2010;18:17322–38.
74. Turkevich J. Colloidal gold - Part II. Gold Bull 1985;18:125.
75. Liz-Marzan L. Tailoring surface plasmons through the morphology and assembly of metal nanoparticles. Langmuir 2006;22:32–41.
76. Link S, El-Sayed M. Spectral properties and relaxation dynamics of surface plasmon electronic oscillations in gold and silver nanodots and nanorods. J Phys Chem B 1999;103:8410–26.
77. Burda C, Chen X, Narayanan R, et al. Chemistry and properties of nanocrystals of different shapes. Chem Rev 2005;105:1025–102.
78. El-Sayed M. Some interesting properties of metals confined in time and nanometer space of different shapes. Acc Chem Res 2001;34:257–64.
79. Jain P, Lee K, El-Sayed I, et al. Calculated absorption and scattering properties of gold nanoparticles of different size, shape, and composition: applications in biological imaging and biomedicine. J Phys Chem B 2006;110:7238–48.
80. Li H, Rothberg L. Colorimetric detection of DNA sequences based on electrostatic interactions with unmodified gold nanoparticles. Proc Natl Acad Sci U S A 2004;101:14036–9.
81. Lee H, Joo S, Lee S, et al. Colorimetric genotyping of single nucleotide polymorphism based on selective aggregation of unmodified gold nanoparticles. Biosens Bioelec-tron 2010;26:730–5.
82. Kanjanawarut R, Su X. Colorimetric detection of DNA using unmodified metallic nanoparticles and peptide nucleic acid probes. Anal Chem 2009;81:6122–9.
83. Liu M, Yuan M, Lou X, et al. Label-free optical detection of single-base mismatches by the combination of nuclease and gold nanoparticles. Biosens Bioelectron 2011;26:4294–300.
84. Hurst S, Lytton-Jean A, Mirkin C. Maximizing DNA loading on a range of gold nanoparticle sizes. Anal Chem 2006;78:8313–8.
85. Thaxton C, Georganopoulou D, Mirkin C. Gold nanoparticle probes for the detection of nucleic acid targets. Clin Chim Acta 2006;363:120–6.
86. Sato K, Hosokawa K, Maeda M. Colorimetric biosensors based on DNA-nanoparticle conjugates. Anal Sci 2007;23:17–20.
87. Ogawa A, Maeda M. Simple and rapid colorimetric detection of cofactors of ap-tazymes using noncrosslinking gold nanoparticle aggregation. Bioorg Med Chem Lett 2008;18:6517–20.
88. Cao YC, Jin RC, Mirkin CA. Nanoparticles with Raman spectroscopic fingerprints for DNA and RNA detection. Science 2002;281:1536–40.

89. Huber M, Wei T, Müller UR, et al. Gold nanoparticle probe-based gene expression analysis with unamplified total human RNA. Nucleic Acids Res 2004;32:e137.
90. Liang RQ, Li W, Li Y, et al. An oligonucleotide microarray for microRNA expression analysis based on labeling RNA with quantum dot and nanogold probe. Nucleic Acids Res 2005;33:e17.
91. Baptista P, Doria G, Henriques D, et al. Colorimetric detection of eukaryotic gene expression with DNA-derivatized gold nanoparticles. J Biotechnol 2005;119:111–7.
92. Doria G, Franco R, Baptista P. Nanodiagnostics: fast colorimetric method for single nucleotide polymorphism/mutation detection. IET Nanobiotechnol 2007;1:53–7.
93. Veigas B, Machado D, Perdigão J, et al. Au-nanoprobes for detection of SNPs associated with antibiotic resistance in Mycobacterium tuberculosis. Nanotechnology 2010;21:415101.
94. Costa P, Amaro A, Botelho A, et al. Gold nanoprobe assay for the identification of mycobacteria of the Mycobacterium tuberculosis complex. Clin Microbiol Infect 2010;16:1464–9.
95. Silva LB, Veigas B, Doria G, et al. Portable optoelectronic biosensing platform for identification of mycobacteria from the Mycobacterium tuberculosis complex. Biosens Bioelectron 2011;26:2012–17.
96. Conde J, de la Fuente JM, Baptista PV. RNA quantification using gold nanoprobes - application to cancer diagnostics. J Nanobiotechnology 2010;8:5.
97. Baptista PV, Doria G, Conde J. Alloy metal nanoparticles for multicolor cancer diagnostics. In: Proceeding of SPIE Vol. 7909 79090K-1, SPIE West 2011, Colloidal Quantum Dots/Nanocrystals for Biomedical Applications VI. San Francisco (CA): 2011.
98. Doria G, Larguinho M, Dias JT, et al. Gold-silver-alloy nanoprobes for one-pot multiplex DNA detection. Nanotechnology 2010;21:255101.

# Role of Nanodiagnostics in Personalized Cancer Therapy

Kewal K. Jain, MD, FRACS, FFPM

### KEYWORDS

- Cancer biomarkers • Cancer diagnosis • Nanobiotechnology
- Nanodiagnostics • Nanoparticles • Personalized medicine

*Nanodiagnostics* is the term used for application of nanobiotechnology for molecular diagnosis, which is important for developing personalized cancer therapy. Personalized medicine is the prescription of specific therapeutics best suited for an individual. It is usually based on pharmacogenetic, pharmacogenomic, and pharmacoproteomic information but also takes into consideration environmental factors that influence response to therapy.[1] Combination of diagnostics with therapeutics, an important feature of personalized cancer therapy, is facilitated by the use of nanobiotechnology.[2] Nanodiagnostic technologies are also being used to refine discovery of biomarkers, as nanoparticles offer advantages of high volume/surface ratio and multifunctionality. Biomarkers are important basic components of personalized medicine and are applicable to management of cancer as well.

## NANODIAGNOSTIC TECHNOLOGIES RELEVANT TO CANCER

Early diagnosis of cancer is important for personalized management. Nanobiotechnology will contribute to early detection of cancer as follows:

- It can complement existing technologies and make significant contributions to cancer detection, prevention, diagnosis, and treatment.
- It would be extremely useful in the area of biomarker research and provide additional sensitivity in assays with relatively small sample volumes.

Examples of applications of nanobiotechnology in cancer diagnostics include dendrimers, quantum dots (QDs), gold nanoparticles, and use of nanoparticles for tumor imaging.

### Dendrimers for Sensing Cancer Cell Apoptosis

Poly(amidoamine) (PAMAM) dendrimers have been used as a platform for the targeted delivery of chemotherapeutic drugs in cancer. A PAMAM nanodevice can be

The author has no financial involvement in the topic of the article and there is no conflict of interest.
Department of Biotechnology, Jain PharmaBiotech, Blaesiring 7, Basel 4057, Switzerland
*E-mail address:* jain@pharmabiotech.ch

used to monitor the rate and extent of cell killing, or apoptosis, caused by the delivered chemotherapeutic drug, which is important for predicting clinical efficacy.[3] Whereas other approaches to detect apoptosis rely on the human protein annexin V, which binds to a hidden cell membrane component seen in the initial stages of apoptosis, this method detects caspase-3, an enzyme activated early in the apoptosis process. This enzyme cleaves the bond between 2 specific amino acids, and this specificity has been exploited to design fluorescence resonance energy transfer (FRET)-based assays for caspase-3. The fluorescence appears only when caspase-3 breaks a valine-aspartic acid bond in a specially designed substrate for this enzyme. To create a tumor-specific apoptosis detector, folic acid and the caspase-3 substrate were attached to a PAMAM dendrimer. Folic acid acts as a tumor-targeting agent, binding to folic acid that many types of tumor cells produce in abundance. Apoptotic tumor cells bearing this folic acid receptor take up the dendrimer and fluoresce brightly. In contrast, apoptotic cells lacking the folic acid receptor do not fluoresce.

### Detection of Circulating Cancer Cells

A method has been described for magnetically capturing circulating tumor cells in the bloodstream of mice followed by rapid photoacoustic detection.[4] Magnetic nanoparticles, which were functionalized to target a receptor commonly found in breast cancer cells, bound and captured circulating tumor cells under a magnet. To improve detection sensitivity and specificity, gold-plated carbon nanotubes conjugated with folic acid were used as a second contrast agent for photoacoustic imaging. By integrating in vivo multiplex targeting, magnetic enrichment, signal amplification, and multicolor recognition, this approach enables circulating tumor cells to be concentrated from a large volume of blood in the vessels of tumor-bearing mice and has potential applications for the early diagnosis of cancer and the prevention of metastasis in humans.

### Differentiation Between Normal and Cancer Cells by Nanosensors

Rapid and effective differentiation between normal and cancer cells is an important challenge for the diagnosis and treatment of tumors. A nanoparticle array-based system has been described for identification of normal and cancer cells based on a "chemical nose/tongue" approach that exploits subtle changes in the physicochemical nature of different cell surfaces.[5] Differential interactions with functionalized nanoparticles are transduced through displacement of a multivalent polymer fluorophore that is quenched when bound to the particle and fluorescent after release. This sensing method can rapidly (minutes/seconds) and effectively distinguish between different cell types, such as normal, cancerous, and metastatic human breast cells.

### Gold Nanoparticles for Cancer Diagnosis

Gold nanoparticles conjugated to anti–epidermal growth factor receptor (anti-EGFR) monoclonal antibodies (MAbs) specifically and homogeneously bind to the surface of the cancer cells with 600% greater affinity than to the noncancerous cells. This specific and homogeneous binding is found to give a relatively sharper surface plasmon resonance (SPR) absorption band with a red shifted maximum compared with that observed when added to the noncancerous cells.[6] The particles that worked the best were 35 nm in size. These results suggest that SPR scattering imaging or SPR absorption spectroscopy generated from antibody-conjugated gold nanoparticles can be useful in molecular biosensor techniques for the diagnosis and investigation of living oral epithelial cancer cells in vivo and in vitro. Advantages of this technique are

- It is not toxic to human cells. A similar technique with QDs uses semiconductor crystals to mark cancer cells, but the semiconductor material is potentially toxic to the cells and humans.
- It does not require expensive high-powered microscopes or lasers to view the results. All it takes is a simple, inexpensive microscope and white light.
- Results are instantaneous. If a cancerous tissue is sprayed with gold nanoparticles containing the antibody, the results can be seen immediately. The scattering is so strong that a single particle can be detected.

An animal study has successfully demonstrated the safety of diagnostic use of Raman-silica-gold-nanoparticles (R-Si-Au-NPs), which overcome the inherently weak nature of Raman effect by producing larger Raman signals through surface-enhanced Raman scattering.[7] R-Si-Au-NPs were bound to polyethylene glycol (PEG) molecules to improve biological tolerance. Molecules that home in on cancer cells can be attached to PEG-R-Si-Au-NPs, and the overall diameter is 100 nm. Photoimaging with these nanoparticles holds the promise of very early disease detection in colorectal cancer (CRC), even before any gross anatomic changes show up, without physically removing any tissue from the patient. Both rectal and intravenous administration of the particles did not show any systemic toxicity in experimental animals. Furthermore, the nanoparticles were excreted quickly. The intravenously administered nanoparticles were sequestered rapidly by scavenger cells resident in organs such as the liver and spleen. This opens the door to human tests of intravenous injections of these nanoparticles to search for tumors throughout the body. Molecules targeting breast, lung, or prostate cancer can be attached to these nanoparticles. Clinical studies of the nanoparticles for the diagnosis of CRC are ongoing.

Chemiluminescence resonance energy transfer (CRET) by using gold nanoparticles (AuNPs) has been applied for immunoassay of alpha fetoprotein (AFP)—a biomarker of cancer.[8] The detection limit of AFP was 2.5 ng mL$^{-1}$. The results are in good agreement with enzyme-linked immunosorbent assays. This approach is expected to be extended to other assays using other antibodies, analytes, and chemiluminescent substances.

Melanoma cells are tagged with gold nanoparticles to show increased sensitivity to detection in a photoacoustic system.[9] This technique has the potential to improve detection of circulating tumor cells (CTCs), which are an important prognostic factor in the progress of melanoma. Gold nanoparticles can be heated rapidly whenever exposed to infrared light of the right wavelength. Heating of gold nanoparticles results in variations in pressure surrounding them, which, in turn, is expressed in the generation of ultrasound—a phenomenon called *plasmon resonance*. Highly sensitive detection of cancer cells has been shown using photoacoustic imaging and plasma resonance of gold nanoparticles.

### Gold Nanorods for Detection of Metastatic Tumor Cells

Gold nanorods absorb near-infrared (NIR) frequencies and can be used as multifunctional agents for biological imaging and combination of diagnostics with therapeutics. Gold nanorods can support nonlinear optical microscopy based on 2-photon-excited luminescence and can enhance the contrast of biomedical imaging with optical coherence tomography and photoacoustic tomography.[10] Gold nanorods are also efficient at mediating the conversion of NIR light energy into heat and can generate localized photothermal effects for destroying cancer cells.

An antibody that recognizes one specific cancer cell surface biomarker can be attached to each nanorod of a given length and diameter. A gold nanorod-antibody construct that recognizes a biomarker found on tumor cell surfaces can be used to characterize tumors according to their cellular composition and correlate their findings to the metastatic potential of each given cell type. Gold nanorods can enable monitoring of as many as 15 different antibody-nanorod constructs simultaneously.

## Nanobiosensors for Detection of Cancer

Nanoscale biosensors, or nanobiosensors, provide investigators with an unprecedented level of sensitivity, often to the single molecule level. Lab-on-a-chip devices containing an array of nanobiosensors could be used for rapid screening of small samples of tumor at low cost.[11]

An implantable nanobiosensor that uses a semipermeable membrane to contain nanoparticle magnetic relaxation switches can sense the local in vivo environment and may be left behind during biopsy.[12] A cell line secreting a model cancer biomarker produced ectopic tumors in mice. Magnetic resonance imaging showed that the transverse relaxation time (T2) of devices in tumor-bearing mice was lower than that in devices in control mice. Short-term applications for this device are numerous, including verification of successful tumor resection. The ability to repeatedly sample the local environment for tumor biomarker, chemotherapeutic agent, and tumor metabolite concentrations could improve early detection of metastasis and personalized therapy.

An implant for magnetic sensing for cancer contains nanoparticles that can be designed to test for different substances, including metabolites, such as glucose and oxygen that are associated with tumor growth. It can also be used to test the effects of anticancer drugs in individual patients; the implant could reveal how much of a drug has reached the tumor. The nanoparticles are encased in a silicone delivery device, enabling their retention in patients' bodies for an extended period. The device can be implanted directly into a tumor, allowing a more direct look at what is happening in the tumor over a period of time. The technique makes use of detection nanoparticles composed of iron oxide and coated with dextran. Antibodies specific to the target molecules are attached to the surface of the particles. When the target molecules are present, they bind to the particles and cause them to clump together. That clumping can be detected by magnetic resonance imaging (MRI). The nanoparticles are trapped inside the silicone device, which is sealed off by a porous membrane. The membrane allows molecules smaller than 30 nm to get in, but the detection particles are too large to get out. In addition to monitoring the presence of chemotherapy drugs, the device could also be used to check whether a tumor is growing or shrinking, or whether it has spread to other locations, by sensing the amount and location of tumor biomarkers. Preclinical testing is planned for this device using human chorionic gonadotropin, which can be considered a biomarker for cancer because it is produced by tumors and not normally found in healthy individuals except in pregnant women.

## Single-Wall Carbon Nanotubes for Detection of Cancer Proteins

Single-wall carbon nanotubes (SWCNTs) are being developed for monitoring cancer-specific proteins. These are highly sensitive to single-protein binding events and can be massively multiplexed with millions of tubes per chip for proteomic profiling. The tubes have extraordinary strength, unique electronic properties, and the ability to tag cancer-specific proteins to their surface. These tubes can be fabricated by decomposition of carbon-based gas in a furnace, using iron nanoparticles as catalyst material. With diameter of 1 nm and length of 1 $\mu$m, these tubes are smaller than a single strand of DNA. In other words, this tube is an atomic arrangement of 1 layer of carbon atoms, which are on the surface. Protein binding events occurring on the surface of these nanotubes produce a measurable change in the mechanical and electrical properties.

Coating the surfaces of SWCNTs with MAbs facilitates detection of CTCs in the blood. This method could be used for detection of recurring CTCs or micrometastases remaining from the originally treated tumor. The technique could be cost effective and could diagnose whether cells are cancerous quickly rather than in days required for conventional histology examination. An electrochemical immunosensor has been developed for the detection of matrix metalloproteinase-3, a cancer biomarker, based on vertically aligned SWCNT arrays.[13] This is a rapid, simple, and cost-effective method for screening of the cancer biomarker for point-of-care diagnosis. Electrochemical immunosensors using vertically aligned SWCNT forests can provide ultrasensitive, accurate cancer biomarker protein assays.[14] The reasons for sensitivity can be assigned to the dense packing of carboxylated SWCNT forest tips, which enable a large surface concentration of capture MAbs.

### Nanobiochip Sensor Technique for Analysis of Oral Cancer Biomarkers

A pilot study has described a nanobiochip sensor technique for analysis of oral cancer biomarkers in exfoliative cytology specimens, targeting both biochemical and morphologic changes associated with early oral tumorigenesis.[15] Oral lesions from dental patients, along with normal epithelium from healthy volunteers, were sampled using a noninvasive brush biopsy technique. Specimens were enriched, immunolabeled, and imaged in the nanobiochip sensor according to previously established assays for the EGFR biomarker and cytomorphometry. Four key parameters were significantly elevated in both dysplastic and malignant lesions relative to healthy oral epithelium, including the nuclear area and diameter, the nuclear-to-cytoplasmic ratio, and EGFR biomarker expression. Further examination using logistic regression and receiver operating characteristic curve analyses identified morphologic features as the best predictors of disease individually, whereas a combination of all features further enhanced discrimination of oral cancer and precancerous conditions with high sensitivity and specificity. Further clinical trials are necessary to validate the regression model and evaluate other potential biomarkers. Nanobiochip sensor technique is a promising tool for early detection of oral cancer, which could enhance patient survival.

### Nanodots for Tracking Apoptosis in Cancer

Apoptosis is a hallmark effect triggered by anticancer drugs. A biocompatible, fluorescent nanoparticle has been developed that could provide an early sign that apoptosis is occurring as a result of anticancer therapy.[16] The fluorescent surface-enhanced Raman spectroscopic (F-SERS) nanodots were created to boost the optical signal generated by typical, biocompatible fluorescent dyes. The nanodots consist of silver nanoparticles embedded in a silica sphere. Attached to the silica core are fluorescent dye molecules and molecules known as Raman labels that enhance the electronic interactions between the silver nanoparticles and the dye molecules. The researchers also linked annexin-V, a molecule that binds specifically to a chemical that appears on cells undergoing apoptosis, to the silica-silver nanoparticle construct. Toxicity tests showed that the silica-silver nanodots were not toxic to various human cells growing in culture. The investigators then added the nanodots to cells triggered to undergo apoptosis and were able to image those cells as they went through programmed cell death. Based on these results, the researchers prepared other nanodots containing antibodies that bind to other molecules involved in apoptosis. They then added these antibody-linked nanodots and the annexin V–linked nanodots to cultured human lung cancer cells. The investigators were able to track the appearance of all 3 molecules simultaneously, which has been difficult to do using conventional cell staining techniques.

### Nanolaser Spectroscopy for Detection of Cancer in Single Cells

Nanolaser scanning confocal spectroscopy can be used to identify a previously unknown property of certain cancer cells that distinguishes them with single cell resolution from closely related normal cells.[17] This property is the correlation of light scattering and spatial organization of mitochondria; normally, it is well scattered, but in cancer cells, the mitochondria are disorganized and scatter light poorly. These optical methods are promising powerful tools for detecting cancer at an early stage.

### Nanoparticles Designed for Dual-Mode Imaging of Cancer

The best characteristics of QDs and magnetic iron oxide nanoparticles have been combined to create a single nanoparticle probe that can yield clinically useful images of both tumors and the molecules involved in cancer.[18] Synthetic 30-nm-diameter silica nanoparticles are impregnated with rhodamine, a bright fluorescent dye, and 9-nm-diameter water-soluble iron oxide nanoparticles. These 2 nanoparticles are then mixed with a chemical linker, yielding the dual-mode nanoparticle. On average, 10 magnetic iron oxide particles link to a single dye-containing silica nanoparticle, and the resulting construct is approximately 45 nm in diameter. The combination nanoparticle performed better in both MRI and fluorescent imaging tests than did the individual components. In MRI experiments, the combination nanoparticle generated an MRI signal that was over 3-fold more intense than the same number of iron oxide nanoparticles. Similarly, the fluorescent signal from the dual-mode nanoparticle was almost twice as bright as that produced by dye molecules linked directly to iron oxide nanoparticles. Next, the dual-mode nanoparticles were labeled with an antibody that binds to molecules known as polysialic acids, which are found on the surface of certain nerve cell and lung tumors. These targeted nanoparticles were quickly taken up by cultured tumor cells and were readily visible using fluorescence microscopy.

### Nanotechnology-Based Single Molecule Assays for Cancer

Information about the biological processes in living cells is required for the detection and diagnosis of cancer for the following reasons:

- For recognizing the important changes that occur when cells undergo malignant transformation.
- For situations in which primary cells obtained from a surgical procedure cannot be propagated because of the type of cell or the low number of cells available
- For detection of cancer at an early stage, which is a critical step for improving cancer treatment.

Early detection requires sensitive methods for isolating and interrogating individual cells with high spatial and temporal resolution without disrupting their cellular biochemistry. Probes designed to penetrate a cell and report on the conditions within that cell must be sufficiently small, exceedingly bright, and stable for a long time in the intracellular environment without disrupting the cell's normal biochemical functioning. A series of silver nanoparticles have been prepared that meet many of the criteria listed above.[19] Although smaller than 100 nm in diameter, these particles are bright enough to be seen by the eye using optical microscopy. Unlike fluorophores, fluorescent proteins, or quantum dots, silver nanoparticles do not photodecompose during extended illumination. Therefore, they can be used as a probe to continuously monitor dynamic events in living cells during studies that last for weeks or even months. Because the color of the scattered light from nanoparticles depends on their size, they have been used to measure the change in single membrane pores in real time using dark-field optical microscopy. Intracellular and extracellular nanoparticles can also be differentiated by the intensity of light scattering. The next challenge is to develop methods for modifying the surface of the nanoparticles to make them more biocompatible, so that biological processes can be observed without disturbing or destroying the cell's intrinsic biochemical machinery. Ultimately, these probes may be combined to produce highly sensitive assays with high spatial and temporal resolution. This advance will enable researchers to study the interactions of multiple genes in the same cell simultaneously by using different-colored reporter molecules. In addition to transcription and translation, similar live-cell single molecule assays will offer the prospect of studying more complex cellular processes, such as cell signaling. Continuous advances and evolution along these research fronts are necessary to unravel biochemical processes in vivo and to develop tools that can be used to detect and diagnose cancer using only a single cell from the patient.

### QDs for Detection of Tumors

QD immunofluorescent labeling is useful for imaging of cancer cells. QD bioconjugates that are highly luminescent and stable enable visualization of cancer cells in living animals. An electrochemical cytosensor has been devised by using aptamer-QD conjugates as a platform for tumor cell recognition and detection.[20] Combination of aptamer and nanoparticles can be used for cell analysis, which is important for cancer diagnosis and therapy. Single-domain antibody bioconjugated NIR-QDs have potential for development of optical molecular imaging for early-stage cancer diagnosis.[21]

### QD-Based Test for DNA Methylation

DNA methylation contributes to carcinogenesis by silencing key tumor suppressor genes. An ultrasensitive and reliable nanotechnology assay, MS-qFRET (fluorescence resonance energy transfer) can detect and quantify DNA methylation.[22] Bisulfite-modified DNA is subjected to polymerase chain reaction (PCR) amplification with primers that would differentiate between methylated and unmethylated DNA. QDs are then used to capture PCR amplicons and determine the methylation status via FRET. The specific target of the test is DNA methylation, which occurs when methyl attaches to cytosine, a DNA building block. When this happens at specific gene locations, it can stop the release of tumor-suppressing proteins; cancer cells then more easily form and multiply. The method involves singling out the DNA strands with methyl attachments through bisulfite conversion, whereby all nonmethyl segments are converted into another nucleotide. Copies of the remaining DNA strands are made, 2 molecules (a biotin protein and a fluorescent dye) are attached at either end, and the strands are mixed with QDs that are coated with a biotin-attractive chemical. Up to 60 DNA strands are attracted to a single QD. An ultraviolet light or blue laser activates the QDs, which pass the energy to the fluorescent molecules on the DNA strands, which then light up and are identifiable via a spectrophotometer, which identifies and can count the DNA methylation.

Key features of MS-qFRET include its low intrinsic background noise, high resolution, and high sensitivity. This approach detects as little as 15 pg of methylated DNA in the presence of a 10,000-fold excess of unmethylated alleles, enables reduced use of PCR (as low as eight cycles), and allows for multiplexed analyses. The high sensitivity of MS-qFRET enables 1-step detection of methylation at PYCARD, CDKN2B, and CDKN2A genes in patient sputum samples that contain low concentrations of methylated DNA, which normally would require a nested PCR approach.

The direct application of MS-qFRET on clinical samples offers great promise for its translational use in early cancer diagnosis and prognostic assessment of tumor behavior, as well as monitoring response to therapeutic agents. Gene DNA methylation indicates a higher risk of cancer development and is also seen as a warning sign of genetic mutations that lead to development of cancer. Moreover, because different cancer types possess different genetic markers, eg, lung cancer biomarkers differ from those of leukemia, the test should identify which cancer for which a patient is at risk. This test could be used for frequent screening for cancer and replacing traditionally invasive methods with a simple blood test. It could also help determine whether a cancer treatment is effective and thus enable personalized chemotherapy.

### Nanobiotechnology for Early Detection of Cancer to Improve Treatment

Cancer cells themselves may be difficult to detect at an early stage, but they leave a fingerprint, ie, a pattern of change in biomarker proteins that circulate in the blood. There may be 20 to 25 biomarkers, which may require as many as 500 measurements, all of which should be made from a drop of blood obtained by pinprick. Thus, nanoscale diagnostics will play an important role in this effort. Nanowire biosensors in development at the California Institute of Technology (Pasadena, CA, USA) can electronically detect a few protein molecules along with other biomarkers that are early signs of cancer. Nanowires in a set are coated with different compounds; each of these compounds binds to a particular biomarker and changes the conductivity of the nanowire that can be measured. Thousands of such nanowires are combined on a single microfluidic chip that enables identification of the type of cancer. Currently, such a chip can detect between 20 to 30 biomarkers.

An automated gold nanoparticle bio-barcode assay probe has been described for the detection of prostate-specific antigen (PSA) at 330 fg/mL, along with the results of a clinical pilot study designed to assess the ability of the assay to detect PSA in the serum of 18 men who have undergone radical prostatectomy for prostate cancer.[23] Available PSA immunoassays often are not capable of detecting PSA in the serum of men after radical prostatectomy. This new bio-barcode PSA assay is approximately 300 times more sensitive than commercial immunoassays, and all patients in this study had a measurable serum PSA level after radical prostatectomy. Because the patient outcome depends on the level of PSA, this ultrasensitive assay enables

- Reassurance to the patients, who have undetectable PSA levels with conventional assays, but detectable and nonincreasing levels with the barcode assay, that their cancer will not recur
- Earlier detection of recurrence because of the ability to measure increasing levels of PSA before conventional tests can measure them
- Use of PSA levels, which would otherwise not be detectable with conventional assays, to follow the response of patients to treatment.

### IMPACT OF NANOTECHNOLOGY-BASED IMAGING IN MANAGEMENT OF CANCER

Nanotechnology plays an important role in diagnostic imaging of cancer, particularly by MRI. Nanotechnology-based cancer imaging will lead to sensitive and accurate detection of early-stage cancer and also help in accurate delivery of cancer therapy.

## Cornell Dots for Cancer Imaging

Cornell dots (C dots) are ultrasmall, multimodal silica nanoparticle greater than 7 nm in diameter, which have been surface functionalized with cyclic arginine-glycine-aspartic acid peptide ligands for targeting cancer as well as radioiodine. C dots exhibit high-affinity binding, favorable tumor/blood residence time ratios, and enhanced tumor-selective accumulation in $\alpha v \beta 3$ integrin-expressing melanoma xenografts in mice.[24] The silica shell, essentially glass, is chemically inert and small enough to pass through the body and out in the urine. Coating the dots by PEGylation further protects them from being recognized by the body as foreign substances, giving them more time to find targeted tumors. The outside of the shell can also be coated with organic molecules that can attach to desired targets on tumor surfaces or within tumors. The cluster of dye molecules in a single dot fluoresces under NIR light much more brightly than single dye molecules, and the fluorescence identifies malignant cells, showing a surgeon exactly what needs to be cut out and helping ensure that all malignant cells are found. C dots can reveal the extent of a tumor's blood vessels, cell death, treatment response, and invasive or metastatic spread to lymph nodes and distant organs. The US Food and Drug Administration has approved the first clinical trial in humans of C dots that can light up cancer cells in PET-optical imaging. The technology aims to safely show surgeons the extent of tumors in human organs. The trial is being conducted at Memorial Sloan-Kettering Center, New York. Commercial development will be in collaboration with Hybrid Silica Technologies Inc. (Cambridge, MA, USA).

## Nanoparticle MRI for Tracking Cells in Cancer Therapy

Superparamagnetic iron oxide nanoparticles (SPIONs) can be attached to cells without affecting cell proliferation, differentiation, and function. A clinical study using SPION-labeled dendritic cells was conducted in Europe.[25] Autologous dendritic cells were labeled with a clinical SPION formulation or [111]In-oxine and were co-injected intranodally in melanoma patients under ultrasound guidance. This phase I trial showed the feasibility and safety of imaging intranodal cell trafficking in patients. In contrast to scintigraphic imaging, MRI enables assessment of the accuracy of dendritic cell delivery and of inter- and intranodal cell migration patterns. MRI cell tracking using iron oxides appears clinically safe and well suited to monitor cellular therapy in humans.

Mesenchymal stem cells (MSCs) have the intrinsic ability to home in to growing tumors and can be used as carriers of SPIONs to enable cell tracking and cancer detection as well as simultaneous delivery of gene therapy directly into the tumors.[26] It is believed that MRI cell tracking will become an important technique that someday may become routine in standard radiologic practice once stem cell therapy enters clinical practice.

## Nanoparticle Computed Tomography Scan

Use of nanomaterials for one of the most common imaging techniques, computed tomography (CT), has remained unexplored. Current CT contrast agents are based on small iodinated molecules. They are effective in absorbing x-rays, but nonspecific distribution and rapid pharmacokinetics have rather limited their microvascular and targeting performance. While most of the nanoparticles are designed to be used in conjunction with MRI, bismuth sulfide ($Bi_2S_3$) nanoparticles naturally accumulate in lymph nodes containing metastases and show up as bright white spots in CT images.[27] A polymer-coated $Bi_2S_3$ nanoparticle preparation has been proposed as an injectable CT imaging agent. This preparation shows excellent stability at high concentrations, high x-ray absorption (5-fold better than iodine), very long circulation times (>2 hours) in vivo, and an efficacy/safety profile comparable to or better than iodinated imaging agents. The utility of these polymer-coated Bi2S3 nanoparticles for enhanced in vivo imaging of the vasculature, the liver, and lymph nodes has been demonstrated in mice. These nanoparticles and their bioconjugates are expected to become an important adjunct to in vivo imaging of molecular targets and pathologic conditions. Tumor-targeting agents are now being added to the surfaces of these polymer-coated Bi2S3 nanoparticles.

### QDs Aid Lymph Node Mapping in Cancer

An improved method for performing sentinel lymph node (SLN) biopsy, which depends on illuminating lymph nodes during cancer surgery, has been developed using QDs that emit NIR light, a part of the spectrum that is transmitted through biological tissue with minimal scattering.[28] QDs, rendered soluble by using a polydentate phosphene coating, were injected into live pigs and followed visually to the lymph system just beneath the skin of the animals. The new imaging technique allowed the surgeons to clearly see the target lymph nodes without cutting the animals' skin. SLN mapping is a common procedure used to identify the presence of cancer in a single, "sentinel" lymph node, thus avoiding the removal of a patient's entire lymph system. SLN mapping relies on a combination of radioactivity and organic dyes, but the technique is inexact during surgery, often leading to removal of much more of the lymph system than necessary, causing unwanted trauma. QD technique is a significant improvement over the dye/radioactivity method currently used to perform SLN mapping. The imaging system and QDs allowed the pathologist to focus on specific parts of the SLN that would be most likely to contain malignant cells, if cancer were present.

Different varieties of PEG-coated QDs have been injected directly into tumors in mouse models of human cancer and their course tracked through the skin using NIR fluorescence microscopy to image and map SLNs.[29] In tumors that drained almost immediately to the SLNs, the QDs were confined to the lymphatic system, mapping out the connected string of lymph nodes. This provided easy tagging of the SLNs for pathology, and there was little difference in results among the different QD types used. Examination of the SLNs identified by QD localization showed that at least some contained metastatic tumor foci. The animals used in this study were followed up with for more than 2 years, with no evidence of toxicity, even though QDs could still be observed within the animals. SLN mapping has already revolutionized cancer surgery. NIR QDs have the potential to improve this important technique even further. Because the QDs in the study are composed of heavy metals, which can be toxic, they have not yet been approved for clinical use until safety has been established.

### Role of Nanoparticle-Based Imaging in Oncology Clinical Trials

Currently, CT scans are used as surrogate end points in cancer clinical trials. The size of the tumor gives only limited information about the effectiveness of therapy. New imaging agents could speed the clinical trials process in 2 ways: (1) better imaging data could help oncologists select which therapies to use on a particular patient and (2) increasingly sensitive and specific imaging agents will be able to provide real-time information about whether a therapy is working. Currently, oncologists and their patients must wait months to determine if a given therapy is working. Shorter clinical trials would mean that effective new drugs would reach patients quicker, and ineffective drugs would be dropped from clinical trials sooner, allowing drug discoverers to better focus their efforts on more promising therapies.

## COMBINATION OF DIAGNOSTICS AND THERAPEUTICS FOR CANCER
### Biomimetic Nanoparticles Targeted to Tumors

Nanoparticle-based diagnostics and therapeutics hold great promise because multiple functions can be built into the particles. One such function is an ability to home to specific sites in the body. Biomimetic particles that not only home to tumors, but also amplify their own homing, have been described.[30] The system is based on a peptide that recognizes clotted plasma proteins and selectively homes to tumors, where it binds to vessel walls and tumor stroma. Iron oxide nanoparticles and liposomes coated with this tumor-homing peptide accumulate in tumor vessels, where they induce additional local clotting, thereby producing new binding sites for more particles. The system mimics platelets, which also circulate freely but accumulate at a diseased site and amplify their own accumulation at that site. The self-amplifying homing is a novel function for nanoparticles. The clotting-based amplification greatly enhances tumor imaging, and the addition of a drug carrier function to the particles is envisioned.

### Dendrimer Nanoparticles for Targeting and Imaging Tumors

Dendrimer nanoparticles have been used to entrap metal nanoparticles, a combination that could serve as a potent imaging and thermal therapy agent for tumors if it were not for associated toxicity issues. To eliminate the toxicity associated with dendrimer-metal nanoparticle combinations, methods are being developed for modifying the surface of dendrimers laden with gold nanoparticles. This chemical treatment greatly reduces the toxicity of the hybrid nanoparticle without changing its size. Construction of novel dendrimers with biocompatible components, and the surface modification of commercially available dendrimers by PEGylation, acetylation, glycosylation, and amino acid functionalization have also been proposed to solve the safety problem of dendrimer-based nanotherapeutics.[31] There are several opportunities and challenges for the development of dendrimer-based nanoplatforms for targeted cancer diagnosis and therapy.

### Gold Nanoparticle Plus Bombesin for Imaging and Therapy for Cancer

Bombesin (BBN) peptides have shown high affinity toward gastrin-releasing peptide (GRP) receptors in vivo that are overexpressed in prostate, breast, and small cell lung carcinoma. In vivo studies using gold nanoparticles (AuNPs)-BBN and its radiolabeled surrogate 198AuNP-BBN constructs are GRP-receptor-specific, showing accumulation with high selectivity in GRP-receptor-rich prostate tumors implanted in mice with severe combined immunodeficiency.[32] The intraperitoneal mode of delivery was found to be efficient as AuNP-BBN conjugates showed reduced RES organ uptake with concomitant increase in uptake at tumor targets. The selective uptake of this new generation of GRP-receptor-specific AuNP-BBN peptide analogs have clinical potential in molecular imaging using CT techniques, as the contrast numbers in prostate tumor sites are several-fold higher compared with those of the pretreatment group. They also provide synergistic advantages by combining molecular imaging with therapy of cancer.

### Gold Nanorods for Combined Imaging and Therapy of Cancer

In vitro studies have found that gold nanorods are novel contrast agents for both molecular imaging and photothermal cancer therapy.[33] Nanorods are synthesized and conjugated to anti-EGFR MAbs and incubated in cancer cell cultures. The anti-EGFR antibody-conjugated nanorods bind specifically to the surface of the malignant-type cells with a much higher affinity because of the overexpressed EGFR on the cytoplasmic membrane of the malignant cells. As a result of the strongly scattered red light from gold nanorods in dark field, observed using a laboratory microscope, the malignant cells are clearly visualized and diagnosed from the nonmalignant cells. It is found that, after exposure to continuous red laser at 800 nm, malignant cells require about half the laser energy to be photothermally destroyed than the nonmalignant cells. Thus, both efficient cancer cell diagnostics and selective photothermal therapy can be carried out simultaneously.

### Magnetic Nanoparticles for Imaging As Well As Therapy of Cancer

Tumor-targeting dendrimers contain both imaging agent and therapeutic agent. DNA-linked dendrimer nanocluster platform enables the delivery of drugs, genetic materials, and imaging agents to cancer cells, offering the potential for developing combinatorial therapeutics.[34] A dendrimer linked to a fluorescent imaging agent and paclitaxel can identify tumor cells and kill them simultaneously. Multifunctional nanoparticles are also in development for simultaneous imaging and therapeutic applications.

In ovarian cancer, metastasis occurs when cells slough off the primary tumor and float free in the abdominal cavity. If one could use the magnetic nanoparticles to trap drifting cancer cells and pull them out of the abdominal fluid, it may be possible to predict and perhaps prevent metastasis. With this aim, magnetic cobalt spinel ferrite nanoparticles, which have cobalt-spiked magnetite at their core, were coated with biocompatible polygalacturonic acid and functionalized with ligands specific for targeting expressed EphA2 receptors on ovarian cancer cells.[35] By using such magnetic nanoparticle-peptide conjugates, targeting and extraction of malignant cells were achieved with a magnetic field. The particles, which are just 10 nm or less in diameter, are not magnetic most of the time, but when a magnet is present, they become strongly attracted to it. Targeting ovarian cancer cells with receptor-specific peptide-modified magnetic nanoparticles resulted in cell capture from a flow stream in vitro and from the peritoneal cavity of mice in vivo. Successful removal of metastatic cancer cells from the abdominal cavity and from circulation using magnetic nanoparticle conjugates indicates the feasibility of a dialysislike treatment and may improve long-term survival rates of ovarian cancer patients. This approach can be applied for treating other cancers, such as leukemia, once the receptors on malignant cells are identified and the efficacy of targeting ligands is established. This technique will provide a way to test for and even treat metastatic ovarian cancer. Although the nanoparticles were tested inside the bodies of mice, it is possible to construct an external device that would remove a patient's abdominal fluid, magnetically filter out the cancer cells, and then return the fluid to the body. After surgery for removal of the primary tumor, a patient would undergo such a treatment to remove any residual cancer cells. The researchers are currently developing such a filter and testing it on abdominal fluid from human ovarian cancer patients.

### Nanobialys for Combining MRI with Delivery of Anticancer Agents

Although gadolinium has been the dominant paramagnetic metal for MRI contrast, the recent association of this lanthanide with nephrogenic systemic fibrosis, an untreatable disease, has spawned renewed interest in alternative metals for molecular MRI. Manganese was one of the first examples of a paramagnetic contrast material studied in cardiac and hepatic MRI because of efficient site-specific MR T1-weighted molecular imaging. Similar to $Ca^{2+}$ and unlike the lanthanides, manganese is a natural cellular constituent and often a cofactor for enzymes and receptors. Mangafodipir trisodium, a manganese blood pool agent, has been approved as a hepatocyte-specific contrast agent with transient side effects caused by dechelation of manganese from the linear chelate. A self-assembled, manganese-labeled nanobialys MRI nanoparticle has been developed for combined diagnosis and delivery of a chemotherapeutic agent.[36] The "bialy" shape affords increased stability. Nanobialys nanoparticles have been characterized for targeted detection of fibrin, a major biochemical feature of thrombus. A complementary ability of nanobialys to incorporate anticancer compounds with greater than 98% efficiency and to retain more than 80% of these drugs after infinite sink dissolution point to the potential of this platform technology to combine a therapeutic agent with a diagnostic agent.

### Nanoparticles, MRI and Thermal Ablation of Tumors

Nanostructures with surface-bound ligands can be used for the targeted delivery and ablation of CRC. Normal colonic epithelial cells as well as primary CRC and metastatic tumors all express a unique surface-bound guanylyl cyclase C (GCC), which binds the bacterial heat-stable enterotoxin (ST) – a peptide. This makes GCC a potential target for metastatic tumor ablation using ST-bound nanoparticles in combination with thermal ablation with near-infrared or radiofrequency energy absorption.[37] Furthermore, the incorporation of iron or iron oxide nanoparticles into such structures would provide advantages for MRI.

Gold nanoshell-based, targeted, multimodal contrast agents in the NIR are fabricated and utilized as a diagnostic and therapeutic probe for MRI, fluorescence optical imaging, and photothermal cancer therapy of breast carcinoma cells in vitro.[38] This may enable diagnosis as well as treatment of cancer during 1 hospital visit.

In the future, it may be possible for a patient to be screened for breast cancer using MRI techniques with engineered enhanced ferrites as the MRI contrast agent. Enhanced ferrites are a class of ferrites that are specially engineered to have enhanced magnetic or electrical properties and are created through the use of core-shell morphology. Magnetic nanoparticles are coupled to the radio frequency of the MRI, which converts the radio frequency into heat. If a tumor is detected, the physician could increase the power to the MRI coils, and localized heating would destroy the tumor without damage to the surrounding healthy cells. The only hindrance to the development of enhanced ferrites for 100 megahertz applications is a lack of understanding of the growth mechanisms and synthesis-property relationships of these nanoparticles. By studying the mechanism for the growth of the enhanced ferrites, it will be possible to create shells that help protect the metallic core from oxidation in biologically capable media.

### pH Low-Insertion Peptide Nanotechnology for Detection and Targeted Therapy of Cancer

The pH-selective insertion and folding of a membrane peptide, pH low-insertion peptide (pHLIP), can be used to target acidic tissue in vivo, including acidic foci in tumors. pHLIP nanotechnology is considered a promising approach for mapping areas of elevated acidity in the body. The peptide has 3 states: soluble in water, bound to the surface of a membrane, and inserted across the membrane. At physiologic pH, the equilibrium is toward water, which explains its low affinity for cells in healthy tissue; at acidic pH, the equilibrium shifts toward membrane insertion and tissue accumulation. This peptide acts like a nanosyringe to deliver tags or therapy to cells. Tumors can be detected by labeling pHLIP peptide with Cy5.5 and imaging by use of NIR fluorescence with wavelengths in the range of 700 to 900 nm. In a mouse breast adenocarcinoma model, fluorescently labeled pHLIP detects solid acidic tumors with high accuracy and accumulates in them even at a very early stage of tumor development.[39] The fluorescence signal is stable and is approximately 5 times higher in tumors than in healthy counterpart tissue. Tumor targeting is based on the fact that most tumors, even very small ones, are acidic as a result of the way they grow, which is known as the Warburg effect, named after the winner of the Nobel Prize for this discovery in 1931. Tumors may be treated by attaching and delivering anticancer agents with pHLIP.

### QD Conjugates Combine Cancer Imaging, Therapy, and Sensing

The specificity and sensitivity of a QD-aptamer-doxorubicin (QD-Apt-Dox) conjugate as a targeted cancer imaging, therapy, and sensing system has been demonstrated in vitro.[40] By functionalizing the surface of fluorescent QD with a RNA aptamer, which recognizes the extracellular domain of the prostate-specific membrane antigen, the system is capable of differential uptake and imaging of prostate cancer cells that express the prostate-specific membrane antigen. The intercalation of doxocycline (Dox), an anticancer drug with fluorescent properties, in the double-stranded stem of the aptamer results in a targeted conjugate with reversible self-quenching properties based on a Bi-FRET mechanism. A donor-acceptor model FRET between QD and Dox and a donor-quencher model FRET between Dox and aptamer result when Dox is intercalated within the aptamer. This simple multifunctional nanoparticle system can deliver Dox to the targeted prostate cancer cells and sense the delivery of Dox by activating the fluorescence of QD, which concurrently images the cancer cells.

### Radiolabeled Carbon Nanotubes for Tumor Imaging and Targeting

Single-walled carbon nanotubes (SWCNTs) with covalently attached multiple copies of tumor-specific MAbs, radiometal-ion chelates, and fluorescent probes can target lymphomas and deliver both imaging and therapeutic molecules to these tumors.[41] Each nanotube, which contained approximately 6 antibody molecules and 114 radioactive atoms, proved to be stable in human plasma for at least 96 hours and was able to bind to targeted tumor cells. Most importantly, the chemical linkages binding the radioactive element indium-111 was completely stable in human plasma for the entire 4-day experiment. Tests using a mouse model of human lymphoma showed that such a nanotube construct successfully targeted tumors while avoiding healthy cells. The ability to specifically target tumor with prototype-radiolabeled or fluorescent-labeled, antibody-appended SWCNT constructs was encouraging and suggested further investigation of these as diagnostic combined with drug delivery for cancer.

### Ultrasonic Tumor Imaging and Targeted Chemotherapy by Nanobubbles

Drug delivery in polymeric micelles combined with tumor irradiation by ultrasound results in effective drug targeting, but this technique requires prior tumor imaging. One targeted drug delivery method uses ultrasound scan to image tumors and also releases the drug from nanobubbles into the tumor.[42] Mixtures of drug-loaded polymeric micelles and perfluoropentane nanobubbles stabilized by the same biodegradable block copolymer were used in this study. Upon intravenous injection into mice, Dox-loaded micelles and nanobubbles extravasated selectively into the tumor interstitium, where the nanobubbles coalesced to produce microbubbles. When exposed to ultrasound, the bubbles generated echoes, which made it possible to image the tumor. The sound energy from the ultrasound popped the bubbles, releasing Dox, which enhanced intracellular uptake by tumor cells in vitro to a statistically significant extent relative to that observed with nonsonicated nano-bubbles and nonsonicated micelles and resulted in tumor regression in the mouse model. Thus, multifunctional nanoparticles can act as tumor-targeted drug carriers, long-lasting ultrasound contrast agents, and enhance ultrasound-mediated drug delivery to facilitate personalized cancer therapeutics.

### A Cancer-Killing Device Based on Nanotechnology

It is within the realm of possibility to use molecular tools to design a miniature device that can be introduced in the body, locate and identify cancer cells, and finally destroy them. The device would have a biosensor to identify cancer cells and a supply of anticancer substance that could be released on encountering cancer cells. A small computer could be incorporated to program and integrate the combination of diagnosis and therapy and provide the possibility to monitor the in vivo activities by an external device. Because there is no universal anticancer agent, the computer program could match the type of cancer to the most appropriate agent. Such a device could be implanted as a prophylactic measure in persons who do not have any obvious manifestations of cancer. It would circulate freely and could detect and treat cancer at the earliest stage. Such a device could be reprogrammed through remote control and enable change of strategy if the lesion encountered is other than cancer.

### SUMMARY

Nanobiotechnology has greatly refined the diagnosis of cancer not only by detection of biomarkers and in vitro assays but also by molecular imaging for in vivo diagnosis. The most important advantage of the use of nanoparticles is the opportunity to combine diagnosis with delivery of therapy for cancer. Early detection of cancer, refinement of cancer diagnosis and monitoring of cancer therapy will contribute to the development of personalized therapy of cancer. Rapid advances are taking place in nanobiotechnology, and considerable improvements are expected by its applications to the diagnosis and treatment of cancer.

### REFERENCES

1. Jain KK. Textbook of personalized medicine. New York: Springer; 2009.
2. Jain KK. Handbook of nanomedicine. New York: Humana/Springer; 2008.
3. Myc A, Majoros IJ, Thomas TP, et al. Dendrimer-based targeted delivery of an apoptotic sensor in cancer cells. Biomacromolecules 2007;8:13–8.
4. Galanzha EI, Shashkov EV, Kelly T, et al. In vivo magnetic enrichment and multiplex photoacoustic detection of circulating tumour cells. Nat Nanotechnol 2009;4:855–60.
5. Bajaj A, Miranda OR, Kim IB, et al. Detection and differentiation of normal, cancerous, and metastatic cells using nanoparticle-polymer sensor arrays. Proc Natl Acad Sci U S A 2009;106:10912–6.
6. El-Sayed IH, Huang X, El-Sayed MA. Surface plasmon resonance scattering and absorption of anti-EGFR antibody conjugated gold nanoparticles in cancer diagnostics: applications in oral cancer. Nano Lett 2005;5:829–34.
7. Thakor AS, Luong R, Paulmurugan R, et al. The fate and toxicity of Raman-active silica-gold nanoparticles in mice. Sci Transl Med 2011;3:79ra33.
8. Huang X, Ren J. Gold nanoparticles based chemiluminescent resonance energy transfer for immunoassay of alpha fetoprotein cancer marker. Anal Chim Acta 2011; 686:115–20.

9. McCormack DR, Bhattacharyya K, Kannan R, et al. Enhanced photoacoustic detection of melanoma cells using gold nanoparticles. Lasers Surg Med 2011;43:333–8.

10. Wei A, Leonov AP, Wei Q. Gold nanorods: multifunctional agents for cancer imaging and therapy. Methods Mol Biol 2010;624:119–30.

11. Bellan LM, Wu D, Langer RS. Current trends in nanobiosensor technology. Wiley Interdiscip Rev Nanomed Nanobiotechnol 2011;3:229–46.

12. Daniel KD, Kim GY, Vassiliou CC, et al. Implantable diagnostic device for cancer monitoring. Biosens Bioelectron 2009;24:3252–7.

13. Munge BS, Fisher J, Millord LN, et al. Sensitive electrochemical immunosensor for matrix metalloproteinase-3 based on single-wall carbon nanotubes. Analyst 2010; 135:1345–50.

14. Malhotra R, Papadimitrakopoulos F, Rusling JF. Sequential layer analysis of protein immunosensors based on single wall carbon nanotube forests. Langmuir 2010;26: 15050–6.

15. Weigum SE, Floriano PN, Redding SW, et al. Nano-bio-chip sensor platform for examination of oral exfoliative cytology. Cancer Prev Res 2010;3;518–28.

16. Yu KN, Lee SM, Han JY, et al. Multiplex targeting, tracking, and imaging of apoptosis by fluorescent surface enhanced raman spectroscopic dots. Bioconjug Chem 2007; 18:1155–62.

17. Gourlay PL, Hendricks JK, McDonald AE, et al. Mitochondrial correlation microscopy and nanolaser spectroscopy—new tools for biphotonic detection of cancer in single cells. Technol Cancer Res Treat 2005;4:585–92.

18. Choi J, Jun Y, Yeon S, et al. Biocompatible heterostructured nanoparticles for multimodal biological detection. J Am Chem Soc 2006;128:15982–3.

19. Xu X, Patel R. Imaging and assembly of nanoparticles in biological systems. In: Nalwa HS, editor. Handbook of nanostructured biomaterials and their applications in nanobiotechnology. Valencia (CA): American Scientific Publishers; 2005. p. 435–56.

20. Li J, Xu M, Huang H, et al. Aptamer-quantum dots conjugates-based ultrasensitive competitive electrochemical cytosensor for the detection of tumor cell. Talanta 2011;85:2113–20.

21. Zaman MB, Baral TN, Jakubek ZJ, et al. Single-domain antibody bioconjugated near-IR quantum dots for targeted cellular imaging of pancreatic cancer. J Nanosci Nanotechnol 2011;11:3757–63.

22. Bailey VJ, Easwaran H, Zhang Y, et al. MS-qFRET: a quantum dot-based method for analysis of DNA methylation. Genome Res 2009;19:1455–61.

23. Thaxton CS, Elghanian R, Thomas AD, et al. Nanoparticle-based bio-barcode assay redefines "undetectable" PSA and biochemical recurrence after radical prostatectomy. Proc Natl Acad Sci U S A 2009;106:18437–42.

24. Benezra M, Penate-Medina O, Zanzonico PB, et al. Multimodal silica nanoparticles are effective cancer-targeted probes in a model of human melanoma. J Clin Invest 2011;121:2768–80.

25. de Vries JM, Lesterhuis WJ, Barentsz JO, et al. Magnetic resonance tracking of dendritic cells in melanoma patients for monitoring of cellular therapy. Nat Biotechnol 2005;23:1407–13.

26. Tang C, Russell PJ, Martiniello-Wilks R, et al. Concise review: nanoparticles and cellular carriers—allies in cancer imaging and cellular gene therapy? Stem Cells 2010;28:1686–702.

27. Rabin O, Manuel Perez J, Grimm J. An x-ray computed tomography imaging agent based on long-circulating bismuth sulphide nanoparticles. Nat Mater 2006;5:118–22.

28. Kim S, Lim YT, Soltesz EG, et al. Near-infrared fluorescent type-ii quantum dots for sentinel lymph node mapping. Nat Biotechnol 2004;22:93–7.

29. Ballou B, Ernst LA, Andreko S, et al. Sentinel lymph node imaging using quantum dots in mouse tumor models. Bioconjug Chem 2007;18:389–96.
30. Simberg D, Duza T, Park JH, et al. Biomimetic amplification of nanoparticle homing to tumors. Proc Natl Acad Sci U S A 2007;104:932–6.
31. Cheng Y, Zhao L, Li Y, et al. Design of biocompatible dendrimers for cancer diagnosis and therapy: current status and future perspectives. Chem Soc Rev 2011;40:2673–703.
32. Chanda N, Kattumuri V, Shukla R, et al. Bombesin functionalized gold nanoparticles show in vitro and in vivo cancer receptor specificity. Proc Natl Acad Sci U S A 2010;107:8760–5.
33. Huang X, El-Sayed IH, Qian W, et al. Cancer cell imaging and photothermal therapy in the near-infrared region by using gold nanorods. J Am Chem Soc 2006;128:2115–20.
34. Choi Y, Baker JR Jr. Targeting cancer cells with DNA-assembled dendrimers: a mix and match strategy for cancer. Cell Cycle 2005;4:669–71.
35. Scarberry KE, Dickerson EB, McDonald JF, et al. Magnetic nanoparticle–peptide conjugates for in vitro and in vivo targeting and extraction of cancer cells. J Am Chem Soc 2008;130:10258–62.
36. Pan D, Caruthers SD, Hu G, et al. Ligand-directed nanobialys as theranostic agent for drug delivery and manganese-based magnetic resonance imaging of vascular targets. J Am Chem Soc 2008;130:9186–7.
37. Fortina P, Kricka LJ, Graves DJ, et al. Applications of nanoparticles to diagnostics and therapeutics in colorectal cancer. Trends Biotechnol 2007;25:145–52.
38. Bardhan R, Chen W, Perez-Torres C, et al. Nanoshells with targeted simultaneous enhancement of magnetic and optical imaging and photothermal therapeutic response. Advanced Functional Materials 2009;19:3901–9.
39. Andreev OA, Dupuy AD, Segala M, et al. Mechanism and uses of a membrane peptide that targets tumors and other acidic tissues in vivo. Proc Natl Acad Sci U S A 2007;104:7893–8.
40. Bagalkot V, Zhang L, Levy-Nissenbaum E, et al. Quantum dot-aptamer conjugates for synchronous cancer imaging, therapy, and sensing of drug delivery based on bi-fluorescence resonance energy transfer. Nano Lett 2007;7:3065–70.
41. McDevitt MR, Chattopadhyay D, Kappel BJ, et al. Tumor targeting with antibody-functionalized, radiolabeled carbon nanotubes. J Nucl Med 2007;48:1180–9.
42. Rapoport N, Gao Z, Kennedy A. Multifunctional nanoparticles for combining ultrasonic tumor imaging and targeted chemotherapy. J Natl Cancer Inst 2007;99:1095–106.

# Biomarkers Quantification with Antibody Arrays in Cancer Early Detection

Andrea Gallotta, PhD, Enrico Orzes, PhD, Giorgio Fassina, PhD*

**KEYWORDS**

- Cancer biomarkers • Antibody arrays • Biochip
- Cancer screening

Cancer is the second most common cause of death in the United States, accounting for nearly one of every four deaths, exceeded only by heart disease. Cancer is more treatable when diagnosed at the early stage, and this is particularly relevant for cancers of the breast, cervix, mouth, larynx, colon and rectum, and skin. Moreover, cancers of the cervix, colon, and rectum can be prevented by removal of precancerous tissue. There are two major components of early detection of cancer: education to promote early diagnosis and screening.[1]

Recognizing possible warning signs of cancer and taking prompt action leads to early diagnosis and can have a great impact on the disease. Some early signs of cancer include lumps, sores that fail to heal, abnormal bleeding, persistent indigestion, and chronic hoarseness.

Screening refers to the use of simple tests across a healthy population in order to identify individuals who have disease but do not yet have symptoms. Examples include breast cancer screening using mammography and cervical cancer screening using cytology screening methods including Pap smears. Screening programs should be undertaken only when their effectiveness has been demonstrated, when resources (personnel, equipment, and so forth) are sufficient to cover nearly all of the target group, when facilities exist for confirming diagnoses and for treatment and follow-up of those with abnormal results, and when prevalence of the disease is high enough to justify the effort and costs of screening.[1]

## BIOMARKERS AND THEIR USER IN COMBINATION

Circulating biomarkers represent a simple, noninvasive, promising approach for improving detection, diagnosis, and management of some types of cancer. The screening tool must be sufficiently noninvasive and inexpensive to allow widespread applicability. A

The authors have nothing to disclose.

Xeptagen SpA, Via delle Industrie, 9 - 30175 Marghera, Venice, Italy

* Corresponding author.

*E-mail address:* fassina@xeptagen.com

Clin Lab Med 32 (2012) 33–45

doi:10.1016/j.cll.2011.11.001

0272-2712/12/$ – see front matter © 2012 Elsevier Inc. All rights reserved.

substance secreted by tumor tissues easily and cheaply detectable in biological fluids is, therefore, an ideal biomarker because the cancer is detected specifically and noninvasively. Biomarkers measurement and interpretation could be indirect; for example, measures of immune response or hormonal changes induced by tumors.[2]

Cancer is a diverse disease, and it is unlikely that a single biomarker could detect all patients affected by a particular cancer with high specificity and sensitivity. Indeed, biomarkers, such as prostate-specific antigen (PSA) that purport to have high sensitivity tend to have low specificity. Maintaining high specificity (low false-positive rates) is a high priority for population screening. Even a small false-positive rate translates into a large number of people subjected to unnecessary costly diagnostic procedures and psychological stress. Thus, biomarkers need to be highly specific for cancer, and the use of many different biomarkers will likely be necessary for an overall screening program that is both sensitive and specific. Measurement with equivalent accuracy of elevated levels of more than two biomarkers for a given cancer should provide a much better statistical basis for successful prediction than measurement of a single biomarker. Some biomarkers may be useful for the classification, but when combined with others they may become ineffective if they are highly correlated (overlapping). In a stepwise backward selection method, biomarkers that contribute redundant information should be omitted in order to retain a model that contains only biomarkers that are able to improve the diagnostic accuracy. For example, in hepatocellular carcinoma, biomarker-immunoglobulin M (IgM) complexes (squamous cell carcinoma antigen–IgM [SCCA-IgM] and alpha fetoprotein–IgM [AFP-IgM]) may be combined to improve diagnostic accuracy (**Fig. 1**).[3]

A single biomarker expected for a given cancer may for some biochemical reasons be poorly expressed in a particular patient, but it would be unlikely that an entire panel

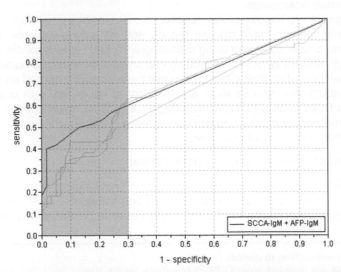

**Fig. 1.** Receiver operating characteristic curves from 60 patients with hepatocellular carcinoma versus 66 cirrhosis donors. The gray area shows the range of specificity between 70% and 100% where partial AUC was calculated ($pAUC_{0.3}$). SCCA-IgM (AUC = 0.689, $pAUC_{0.3}$ = 0.121), AFP-IgM (AUC = 0.632, $pAUC_{0.3}$ = 0.105) and their combination by linear logistic regression (SCCA-IgM + AFP-IgM; AUC = 0.722, $pAUC_{0.3}$ = 0.146). AFP, alpha fetoprotein; AUC, area under curve; IgM, immunoglobulin M; SCCA, squamous cell carcinoma antigen.

of protein biomarkers indicative of that cancer would fail to be expressed. In addition, false-positives and false-negatives may appear frequently with a single biomarker but would be minimized by using a biomarker panel.

Another issue to be considered is that many protein biomarkers are indicative of more than one disease; for example, serum PSA is elevated in some benign prostate diseases as well as prostate cancer. Single cancer biomarkers are often not unique to a specific cancer, but it should be possible to define collections of biomarkers whose elevated individual levels taken together would be reliable predictors for specific cancers.[4]

Detection of panels of biomarkers is further complicated by the fact that ideally both normal and elevated serum levels of biomarkers need to be accurately measured. Ideally, measurements need to be done at high accuracy and cheaply at point of care (POC) such as in a physician's office or clinic to reduce costs, minimize sample decomposition, facilitate on-the-spot diagnosis, and alleviate patient stress. Such POC can also help to guide therapy, especially when timely adjustments in treatment become critical. Given these realities, development of POC bioanalytical devices to measure multiple cancer biomarkers presents a discouraging challenge, but one that nevertheless should be realizable.

In this article the focus is on planar antibody arrays, a possible answer for these POC devices. Antibody arrays are a specific form of protein microarrays in which captured antibodies are spotted and fixed on a solid surface for the purpose of detecting antigens in cancer early detection. The theoretical background for protein microarray-based ligand binding assays was initially developed by Ekins[5] in the late 1980s. According to the model, antibody microarrays not only would permit simultaneous screening of an analyte panel but would also be more sensitive and rapid than conventional screening methods.[5]

## ANTIBODY ARRAYS

Antibody arrays consist of miniaturized devices in which antibodies can be immobilized to capture and quantify specific proteins. One of the main advantages of this technology is the ability to measure hundreds of proteins (biomarkers) using low sample volumes of both precious clinical or biological material and expensive antibodies.[6-8] Understanding the biological events that occur during progression from a normal tissue to cancer and the evidence to use many biomarkers to improve diagnostic accuracy regarding tumors has provided the stimulus to sustain biomarker discovery activities and efforts to evaluate their combination.

As shown in **Fig. 2** and summarized in **Table 1**, several biomarker combinations are suggested for many different tumors. Breast, prostate, and colorectal cancers are the main cancers studied.

## TECHNOLOGICAL OVERVIEW

The high versatility of the design and format of planar antibody arrays has led to multiple versions, and their classification is related to antibody surface, printing methods, labeling, and detection methods.

### Antibody Surface

Immobilization of the antibodies can be performed on planar surfaces such as filter supports, microtiter plates, or glass slides, leading to planar arrays.[5-8] As illustrated in **Box 1**, the two main surfaces used to develop antibody arrays are amorphous material (glass and plastic) and nitrocellulose.

## Antibody Array according to Type of Cancer

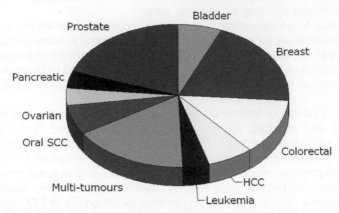

**Fig. 2.** Antibody array according to type of cancer. HCC, hepatocellular carcinoma; SCC, squamous cell carcinoma.

The surface properties of the substrate play an important role in the orientation and conformation of the biomolecule on printed microarray. This orientation is of crucial importance for the functional properties of the biomolecule, the sensitivity of the device, and, hence, on the quality of the applications developed.

### Printing Methods

The antibody must be deposited as microspots in specified positions on the chip. Antibody matrix technology is based mainly on microcontact printing or ink-jet technology (**Box 2**).

Microcontact printing is a form of soft lithography that uses the relief patterns on a master polydimethylsiloxane stamp to form patterns. Advantages of this technique are the simplicity and ease of creating patterns with microscale features, the ability for the array to be created from a single master, the fact that individual stamps can be used several times with minimal degradation of performance, and the fact that this method is inexpensive to fabricate.[47]

Ink-jet technology is a noncontact microdispensing system that allows printing of antibodies on various substrates (nitrocellulose, polystyrene, glass, epoxy, carboxyl, amine, hydrogel). Not all of these surfaces may be treated with contact methods. With ink-jet technology, it is easier to control the antibody amount deposited on each spot, a very important characteristic for developing in vitro diagnosis with high reproducibility. Moreover, with ink-jet technology the minimum amount of antibody deposited for each spot is much less than contact methods (nanoliters vs microliters).[48]

### Labeling and Detection Methods

**Fig. 3** summarizes capture methods and label types of planar antibody arrays.[6–8,49]
Capture methods of antibody arrays comprise the following:

1. *Label-based (one-antibody assays).* The targeted proteins are captured by an immobilized antibody and detected through labeling with a tag.
2. *Sandwich (two-antibody assays).* Immobilized antibodies capture unlabeled proteins, which are detected by another antibody using several methods to generate the signal for detection.

**Table 1**
**Tumors and most often-used markers for screening**

| Type of Cancer | Marker |
|---|---|
| **Colorectal Cancer** | |
| | Apoptotic factors[9] |
| | Various antigens[10–12] |
| **Breast Cancer** | |
| | CA15-3, CEA, HER2, MMP9 and uPA[13] |
| | CA 15-3, EGFR[14] |
| | IL-8[15] |
| | Cytokines and chemochines[16] |
| | HGF[17] |
| | Various antigens[18] |
| **Prostate Cancer** | |
| | AMACR[19] |
| | IL-6, PSA[20] |
| | anti-huTSP1[21] |
| | PSA, PSMA, IL-6, PF-4[22] |
| | PSA, IL-6[23] |
| | Various antibodies[24] |
| **Oral Squamous Cell Carcinoma** | |
| | EGFR[25] |
| | Various antibodies[26] |
| **Hepatocarcinoma** | |
| | AFP, ANG[27] |
| | Apoptotic factors[28] |
| **Leukemia** | |
| | 3D9, 6A5, 4D9,2D5[29] |
| **Ovarian Cancer** | |
| | Various antigens[30] |
| **Pancreatic Cancer** | |
| | Various antigens[31] |
| **Bladder Cancer** | |
| | Cytokines[32] |
| **Multitumors** | |
| | CA125, CA15-3, CA19-9, CA242, CEA, AFP, PSA, fPSA, HGH, beta-HCG, NSE and ferritin[33] |
| | p-Tyr antibodies[34] |
| | AFP, CEA, CA19-9, CA15.3, CA125, b-HCG[35] |
| | AFP, PSA, CRP[36] |
| | Various antigens[37] |

(continued on next page)

| Table 1 (continued) | |
|---|---|
| Type of Cancer | Marker |
| Other[a] | |
| | CRP, CEA[38] |
| | CA19-9, CA125[39] |
| | CEA, CA125, Her-2/Neu (C-erbB-2)[40] |
| | CEA, AFP[41] |
| | CEA[42] |
| | PSA, PSMA, PF-4 and IL-6[43] |
| | Various antigens[44] |

*Abbreviations:* AMACR, Alpha-methylacyl-CoA racemase; ANG, angiogenin; CA, cancer antigen; CEA, anticarcinoembryonic antigen; CRP, C-reactive protein; EGFR, epidermal growth factor receptor; fPSA, free prostate-specific protein; HCG, human chorionic gonadotropin, HER, human epidermal growth factor; HGF, hepatocyte growth factor; HGH, human growth hormone; hu-TSP, human testis-specific protein; IL, interleukin; MMP, matrix metalloproteinase; NSE, neuron-specific enolase; PF, platelet factor; PSA, prostate-specific antigen; PSMA, prostate-specific membrane antigen; p-TYR, phosphotyrosine; uPA, urokinase plasminogen activator.

[a] Tumor not defined.

Label types comprise the following:

1. *Direct labeling.* Proteins/biomarkers (for label-based assays) or secondary antibody (for sandwich assays) are labeled with a fluorophore such as cyanine family (Cy3 or Cy5), quantum dots (QDs) or with an enzyme such as horseradish peroxidase (HRP) in sandwich labeling.

| Box 1 |
|---|
| Types of surfaces used for antibody arrays |
| **Amorphous material— glass and plastic slides** |
| Superaldehyde slides[9,18] |
| Poly(methyl methacrylate) substrate[44] |
| Aminosilanated slides[17,36,38] |
| Polydimethylsiloxane chip[14,26] |
| Silicon chip[21,41] |
| **Nitrocellulose slides** |
| Nitrocellulose[15,18,25,32,33] |
| PATH slides (Gentel)[22,45] |
| FAST slides (Whatman)[12,26,28] |
| **Hydrogels** |
| Hydrogels pads on slide[16,30,34] |
| **Other** |
| Gold-patterned microarray chip[23,27] |

---

**Box 2**
**Biomarker printing methods**

**Ink-Jet**

Packard BioChip Arrayer (PerkinElmer)[16,40]

ScanArray Lite microarray scanner (Packard Bioscience)[19]

PixSys 5000 robot (Cartesian)[17]

Nanoarrayer[21]

GT5000 Gantry System (Cartesian)[33]

PROSYS 7500° (Cartesian)[35]

Microgrid microarraying robot printed (BioRobotics)[37]

**Contact**

GMS 417 microarray printer (Genetic Microsystems Affymetrix)[13,20,26]

VersArray chip writerTM (Bio-Rad)[42]

Proteogen CM-1000 (Proteogen)[38]

Biochip Arrayer (PerkinElmer Life & Analytical Sciences)[22,31,44,45]

M365 syringe pump (Sage)[29]

Polybutadiene PAP pens (Sigma-Aldrich)[46]

**Other**

Hand spotted[9,36]

Photoresist coating[27]

---

2. *Indirect labeling*. Proteins/biomarkers (for label-based assays) or secondary antibody (for sandwich assays) are conjugated with a tag (such as biotin) that is later detected by a second labeled tag (such as streptavidin-HRP, streptavidin-fluorophore, or rolling circle). This approach is an amplification protocol and improves the sensitivity.

Direct label-based assays allow the incubation of two different samples, each labeled with a different tag on the arrays. This type of assay allows the use of a reference sample to be coincubated with a test sample and facilitates normalization. Another benefit is that these assays are competitive, because the analytes in the test and reference solutions compete for binding with the antibodies. This attribute leads to improvement in linearity of response and dynamic range compared with noncompetitive assays. The main disadvantage is related to the disruption of the analyte-antigen interaction by the label, which may also limit the detection as well as the sensitivity and specificity. Moreover, the sample must be treated before introduction into the array, which limits the capability to develop a useful POC device.

The sandwich format increases the specificity compared with label-based assays and reduced background with increasing the sensitivity. This method only allows noncompetitive assays, because only one sample can be incubated on each array. This technique results in a sigmoidal binding response compared with the linear one in the competitive format and requires standard curves of known concentrations of analytes to achieve accurate calibration of concentrations. Compared with label-based assays, the weakness of sandwich assays is the availability of pairs of antibodies for

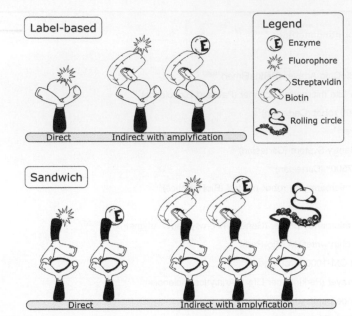

**Fig. 3.** Label-based and sandwich capture methods of planar antibody arrays with different label types.

each antigens and the potential cross-reactivity among detection antibodies increasing with additional analytes. This weakness contrasts with one-antibody assays in which only the availability of antibodies and space on the substrate limit the number of targets analyzed.

Commonly used labels for the visualization/quantification of biomarkers include mainly fluorophores (Cy3, Cy5, QDs, and so forth) and enzymes (alkaline phosphatase, HRP, and so forth).

Detection is by fluorescence or chemiluminescence (**Box 3**). Fluorescence detection is based on the use of fluorochromes that emit light when excited by light of a shorter wavelength. In chemiluminescence, when a soluble organic substrate is applied, the enzyme reacts with the substrate to generate light localized to the sites of enzyme. Chemiluminescence detection is more sensitive than fluorescence, but it requires more incubation and blocking steps.

### Sensitivity and Specificity

Sensitivity and specificity are key parameters for quality and critical steps for the development of antibody array devices. Typical detection range of antibody array has been reported from some picograms to nanograms and usually is better than established enzyme-linked immunoabsorbent assay.[24,49]

Ideally, only the protein of interest reacts with its corresponding binding partner on the microchip. Nonspecific binding may lead to false-positives, rendering protein microchip measurements inaccurate. The potential problem of specificity in the case of antibody microchips is antibodies that interact with multiple proteins. The main causes of this problem are cross-reactivity and multispecificity. Cross-reactivity is the tendency of an antibody to react with an antigen that did not stimulate its production.

---

**Box 3**
**Biomarker detection systems**

**Chemiluminescence**

HRP[15,23,33,46]

BCIP/NBT[18,26]

Electrochemiluminescence[14,32]

**Fluorescence**

Cyanine (Cy3,Cy5) [9,10,17,19,20,22,24,28,30,31,34,36,44,45]

Alexa Fluors[12,21,24,41,43]

Texas Red[16]

Fluorescein isothiocyanate[29,35]

Dyomics (Dy-549, Dy-649)[37]

*Abbreviation:* BCIP/NBT, 5-bromo-4-chloro-3-isdolylphosphate/nitro blue tetrazolium.

---

Multispecificity is a phenomenon when the same antibody reacts with two very different antigens. Both may lead to false-positives.

In label-based direct array, the main disadvantage of antibody array is the disruption of the analyte-antigen interaction by the label, which may limit detection as well as sensitivity and specificity. Moreover, because antibodies cannot be manufactured with preselected affinity and specificity, array sensitivity is antibody-dependent. It is advisable to validate the specificity and sensitivity of each antibody before using it as a probe for antibody arrays.[6,24]

Sensitivity enhancement could be achieved by signal amplification using rolling circle amplification (RCA). In fact, with RCA it is possible to detect 0.1 pg/mL of protein, but this technology requires extensive chemical labeling of the detection antibody and is not easily adaptable in all laboratories.[17,45] An alternative is to use an enzymatic signal enhancement method known as tyramide signal amplification, with which sub-pg/mL levels of protein may be detected.[17]

Reducing background is important to increase the sensitivity. The choices of antibodies and substrates used to develop the device and the step solution applied to treat the array play a key role.

Sensitivity of the microarray could be improved just by minimizing nonspecific binding using washing steps.[23] Another method to reduce background is to develop an alternative microarray using monoclonal antibodies or F(ab')$_2$ fragments as capture probes.[35]

Wang and colleagues[16] show the importance of substrate; in fact, while the nitrocellulose-coated slide performs similar to HydroGel-coated slides at the higher target concentrations, its sensitivity is much lower because of high levels of inherent fluorescent background. Moreover, Lee and colleagues[38] show that the high detection sensitivity can be attributed to the improved surface chemistry of protein immobilization by the bifunctional affinity linker. It is thus proposed that most antibody molecules immobilized are in the correct orientation resulting in increased detection sensitivity.[38]

### *Reproducibility*

Reproducibility (or precision) is the degree to which repeated measurements of the same sample will show the same or similar results. High reproducibility is fundamental to correctly assess the protein quantity and is essential to develop devices for clinical application. Each step in the preparation of an antibody array contributes to generating noise that can affect its reproducibility. Usually, measurements are affected by an error that makes repeated measurements differ from each other. Given a set of measurements, the precision is usually measured by the coefficient of variation (CV; the standard deviation divided by the mean). The precision determined at each concentration level should not exceed 15% of CV except for the lower limit of quantification, where it should not exceed 20%. For high levels of reproducibility, a CV less than 10% on a minimum of three concentrations in the range of expected concentrations is usually considered. Moreover, reproducibility of the system should be evaluated both from an intraassay and interassay approach.[50]

## Stability

Another important aspect for the development of antibody arrays is the stability of the device. Thus, the storage stability of the immunosensor array should be adequate for practical use in order to propose biochips as suitable for clinical diagnostics.

All components of the device should be tested for stability in order to define the shelf life, but the conformational stability of antibody is the most important issue for the reliable detection of biomarkers with microchip-based approaches.

Antibody recognition against protein site (epitope) is dependent on hydrogen bonds, hydrophobic interactions, electrostatic forces, and van der Waals forces. The two- and three-dimensional antibody structure is necessary for binding. Printing methods and arrays surface are the most critical aspects affecting antibody stability. In addition, changes of structure that influence epitope recognition can be caused by an altered reaction environment such as pH, salt concentration, hydrophobicity, or by analysis-related artifacts that are generated during sample processing. Even partially degraded spotted antibodies may bind their corresponding proteins, resulting in decreased signal intensity with consequent quantification errors and/or increases in the coefficients of variation. Manufacturing, storage, and shipping are critical points to maintain the declared stability parameters.

The antibody array stability may vary considerably, depending on different storage times and conditions.[29] Stability may be increased by storing devices in dry air at 4°C.[40]

In stability tests of oriented immobilized antibody, it was found that the antibody array was stable without loss of activity for more than 3 months at 47°C.[38] The advantages of the oriented immobilization of proteins are the good steric accessibility of the active binding site and the increased stability.[36] In addition, stability tests could be used to select the surface and to define the best conditions for the oriented immobilization of antibodies.

## SUMMARY

The aging process in our society will become one of the key driving forces of change over the next decades. The specific demands of older generations constitute a key market of the future, and the pressure to improve and expand health services increases, especially as far as chronic diseases such as cancer are concerned. Availability of efficient and cost-effective screening devices for early detection of cancer are urgently needed to improve quality of life. Mass screening for early detection of cancer will reduce the ever-increasing social costs associated with treating patients with advanced-stage disease where existing diagnostic procedures have failed or screening has been inadequate for broad use. Nanosized technological platforms are the answer for mass screening, especially in those cases in which many different biomarkers need to be determined simultaneously to provide clinical significance even in a decentralized fashion (POC testing). Because biochips automate highly repetitive laboratory tasks by replacing cumbersome equipment with miniaturized assay chemistries, they are able to provide ultrasensitive detection methodologies at significantly lower cost per assay than traditional methods in a significantly smaller amount of space. Biomarkers selection is a key factor for biochip design, in addition to managing the many variables that afflict an array experiment such as instrumental and biological error, reproducibility, array data processing, and normalization.

## REFERENCES

1. American Cancer Society. Cancer Facts & Figures 2011. Atlanta (GA): American Cancer Society; 2011.
2. Huijbers A, Velstra B, Dekker TJ, et al. Proteomic serum biomarkers and their potential application in cancer screening programs. Int J Mol Sci 2010;11:4175–93.
3. Gallotta A, Pengo P, Beneduce L, et al. Factors affecting biochip design for cancer early detection. NanotecIT 2008;10:33–7.
4. Lilja H, Ulmert D, Vickers AJ. Prostate-specific antigen and prostate cancer: prediction, detection and monitoring [review]. Nat Rev Cancer 2008;8(4):268–78[erratum: in: Nat Rev Cancer 2008;8:403].
5. Ekins RP. Ligand assays: from electrophoresis to miniaturized microarrays. Clin Chem 1998;44:2015–30.
6. Sanchez-Carbayo M. Antibody arrays: technical considerations and clinical applications in cancer. Clin Chem 2006;52:1651–9.
7. Haab BB, Dunham MJ, Brown PO. Protein microarrays for highly parallel detection and quantitation of specific proteins and antibodies in complex solutions. Genome Biol 2001;2:RESEARCH0004.
8. Kingsmore SF. Multiplexed protein measurement: technologies and applications of protein and antibody arrays. Nat Rev Drug Discov 2006;5:310–21.
9. Sreekumar A, Nyati MK, Varambally S, et al. Profiling of cancer cells using protein microarrays: discovery of novel radiation-regulated proteins. Cancer Res 2001;61: 7585–93.
10. Madoz-Gúrpide J, Cañamero M, Sanchez L, et al. A proteomics analysis of cell signaling alterations in colorectal cancer. Mol Cell Proteomics 2007;6:2150–64.
11. Zhou J, Belov L, Huang PY, et al. Surface antigen profiling of colorectal cancer using antibody microarrays with fluorescence multiplexing. J Immunol Methods 2010;355: 40–51.
12. Chen C, Chen LQ, Yang GL, et al. The application of C12 biochip in the diagnosis and monitoring of colorectal cancer: systematic evaluation and suggestion for improvement. J Postgrad Med 2008;54:186–90.
13. Luo W, Pla-Roca M, Juncker D. Taguchi design-based optimization of sandwich immunoassay microarrays for detecting breast cancer biomarkers. Anal Chem 2011; 83:5767–74.
14. Du Z, Cheng KH, Vaughn MW, et al. Recognition and capture of breast cancer cells using an antibody-based platform in a microelectromechanical systems device. Biomed Microdevices 2007;9:35–42.
15. Lin Y, Huang R, Chen L, et al. Identification of interleukin-8 as estrogen receptor-regulated factor involved in breast cancer invasion and angiogenesis by protein arrays. Int J Cancer 2004;109:507–15.
16. Wang CC, Huang RP, Sommer M, et al. Array-based multiplexed screening and quantitation of human cytokines and chemokines. J Proteome Res 2002;1:337–43.

17. Woodbury RL, Varnum SM, Zangar RC. Elevated HGF levels in sera from breast cancer patients detected using a protein microarray ELISA. J Proteome Res 2002;1: 233–7.

18. Song XC, Fu G, Yang X, et al. Protein expression profiling of breast cancer cells by dissociable antibody microarray (DAMA) staining. Mol Cell Proteomics 2008;7:163–9.

19. Sreekumar A, Laxman B, Rhodes DR, et al. Humoral immune response to alpha-methylacyl-CoA racemase and prostate cancer. J Natl Cancer Inst 2004;96:834–43 [erratum in: J Natl Cancer Inst 2004;96:1112].

20. Nettikadan S, Radke K, Johnson J, et al. Detection and quantification of protein biomarkers from fewer than 10 cells. Mol Cell Proteomics 2006;5:895–901.

21. Shafer MW, Mangold L, Partin AW, et al. Antibody array profiling reveals serum TSP-1 as a marker to distinguish benign from malignant prostatic disease. Prostate 2007; 67:255–67.

22. Chikkaveeraiah BV, Bhirde A, Malhotra R, et al. Single-wall carbon nanotube forest arrays for immunoelectrochemical measurement of four protein biomarkers for prostate cancer. Anal Chem 2009;81:9129–34.

23. Chikkaveeraiah BV, Mani V, Patel V, et al. Microfluidic electrochemical immunoarray for ultrasensitive detection of two cancer biomarker proteins in serum. Biosens Bioelectron 2011;26:4477–83.

24. Miller JC, Zhou H, Kwekel J, et al. Antibody microarray profiling of human prostate cancer sera: antibody screening and identification of potential biomarkers. Proteomics 2003;3:56–63.

25. McDevitt J, Weigum SE, Floriano PN, et al. A new bio-nanochip sensor aids oral cancer detection. SPIE Newsroom 2011.

26. Knezevic V, Leethanakul C, Bichsel VE, et al. Proteomic profiling of the cancer microenvironment by antibody arrays. Proteomics 2001;1:1271–8.

27. Lee M, Lee S, Lee JH, et al. Highly reproducible immunoassay of cancer markers on a gold-patterned microarray chip using surface-enhanced Raman scattering imaging. Biosens Bioelectron 2011;26:2135–41.

28. Tannapfel A, Anhalt K, Häusermann P, et al. Identification of novel proteins associated with hepatocellular carcinomas using protein microarrays. J Pathol 2003;201:238–49.

29. Du W, Xu Z, Ma X, et al. Biochip as a potential platform of serological interferon alpha2b antibody assay. J Biotechnol 2003;106:87–100.

30. Loch CM, Ramirez AB, Liu Y, et al. Use of high density antibody arrays to validate and discover cancer serum biomarkers. Mol Oncol 2007;1:313–20.

31. Ingvarsson J, Wingren C, Carlsson A, et al. Detection of pancreatic cancer using antibody microarray-based serum protein profiling. Proteomics 2008;8:2211–9.

32. Ghoniem G, Faruqui N, Elmissiry M, et al. Differential profile analysis of urinary cytokines in patients with overactive bladder. Int Urogynecol J 2011;22:953–61.

33. Sun Z, Fu X, Zhang L, et al. A protein chip system for parallel analysis of multi-tumor markers and its application in cancer detection. Anticancer Res 2004;24:1159–65.

34. Gembitsky DS, Lawlor K, Jacovina A, et al. A prototype antibody microarray platform to monitor changes in protein tyrosine phosphorylation. Mol Cell Proteomics 2004;3: 1102–18.

35. Song S, Li B, Wang L, et al. A cancer protein microarray platform using antibody fragments and its clinical applications. Mol Biosyst 2007;3:151–8.

36. Oh SW, Moon JD, Lim HJ, et al. Calixarene derivative as a tool for highly sensitive detection and oriented immobilization of proteins in a microarray format through noncovalent molecular interaction. FASEB J 2005;19:1335–7.

37. Schröder C, Jacob A, Tonack S, et al. Dual-color proteomic profiling of complex samples with a microarray of 810 cancer-related antibodies. Mol Cell Proteomics 2010;9:1271–80.
38. Lee Y, Lee EK, Cho YW, et al. ProteoChip: a highly sensitive protein microarray prepared by a novel method of protein immobilization for application of protein-protein interaction studies. Proteomics 2003;3:2289–304.
39. Sanchez-Carbayo M. Antibody array-based technologies for cancer protein profiling and functional proteomic analyses using serum and tissue specimens. Tumour Biol 2010 31:103–12.
40. Wu J, Zhang Z, Fu Z, et al. A disposable two-throughput electrochemical immunosensor chip for simultaneous multianalyte determination of tumor markers. Biosens Bioelectron 2007;23:114–20.
41. Jokerst JV, Raamanathan A, Christodoulides N, et al. Nano-bio-chips for high performance multiplexed protein detection: determinations of cancer biomarkers in serum and saliva using quantum dot bioconjugate labels. Biosens Bioelectron 2009; 24:3622–9.
42. Hu W, Liu Y, Yang H, et al. ZnO nanorods-enhanced fluorescence for sensitive microarray detection of cancers in serum without additional reporter-amplification. Biosens Bioelectron 2011;26:3683–7.
43. Liu Y, Guo CX, Hu W, et al. Sensitive protein microarray synergistically amplified by polymer brush-enhanced immobilizations of both probe and reporter. J Colloid Interface Sci 2011;360:593–9.
44. Sardesai NP, Barron JC, Rusling JF. Carbon nanotube microwell array for sensitive electrochemiluminescent detection of cancer biomarker proteins. Anal Chem 2011; 83:6698–703.
45. Orchekowski R, Hamelinck D, Li L, et al. Antibody microarray profiling reveals individual and combined serum proteins associated with pancreatic cancer. Cancer Res 2005;65:11193–202.
46. Huang CS, George S, Lu M, et al. Application of photonic crystal enhanced fluorescence to cancer biomarker microarrays. Anal Chem 2011;83:1425–30.
47. Gonzalez-Macia L, Morrin A, Smyth MR, et al. Advanced printing and deposition methodologies for the fabrication of biosensors and biodevices. Analyst 2010;135: 845–67.
48. McWilliam I, Chong Kwan M, Hall D. Inkjet printing for the production of protein microarrays. Methods Mol Biol 2011;785:345–61.
49. Crowther JR. ELISA. Theory and practice. Methods Mol Biol 1995;42:1–218.
50. US Food and Drug Administration. Guidance for industry: bioanalytical method validation. Rockville (MD): US Food and Drug Administration; 2001.

# Cancer Biomarker Detection by Surface Plasmon Resonance Biosensors

Panga Jaipal Reddy, MSc, PhD, Sudipta Sadhu, BTech, MTech,
Sandipan Ray, MSc, PhD, Sanjeeva Srivastava, PhD*

**KEYWORDS**

• Cancer biomarker • Surface plasmon resonance
• Cancer inhibitors • Protein microarray • SPR imaging

Diagnosis of cancer at an early stage of development is essential for effective treatment to control its progression and reduce the mortality rate. Biomarkers are useful candidates for disease diagnosis, monitoring disease progression, and following prognosis in response to the therapeutic interventions.[1–3] Over the last decade there has been a growing interest in analysis of various biological fluids to identify panels of protein markers for cancer, leading to the discovery of several potential targets.[4,5] Despite the sincere efforts from various research groups from all over the world, only a handful of the identified candidates has been approved by the US Food and Drug Administration, which indicates serious "bottle neck" between the "bench-side" findings and their successful "bed-side" implications.[6,7] Multiple issues associated with candidate markers, such as very low abundance, ambiguity, lack of specificity, enormous variation among individuals, and paucity of reproducibility, are hindering their successful translation in clinics.[3,8]

Several proteomic approaches, such as mass spectrometry-based assays,[9] gel-based profiling,[10] and, more recently, protein and antibody arrays,[11] are emerging rapidly as advanced platforms for cancer biomarker discovery and have enhanced our understanding of biological networks at the functional level to provide some mechanistic insight into this fatal disease. However, limited dynamic range and low sensitivity are the major limitations for most of the existing gel and MS-based proteomic approaches.[12] Moreover, accurate diagnosis of complex diseases like cancer requires the simultaneous detection of multiple biomarkers, stipulating the need for high-throughput (HT) detection platforms. To this end, array-based approaches, such as antibody, reverse phase, and functional microarrays, are promising

The authors have nothing to disclose.
Wadhwani Research Center for Biosciences and Bioengineering, Department of Biosciences and Bioengineering, Indian Institute of Technology Bombay, Powai, Mumbai 400076, India
* Corresponding author.
*E-mail address:* sanjeeva@iitb.ac.in

Clin Lab Med 32 (2012) 47–72
doi:10.1016/j.cll.2011.11.002
0272-2712/12/$ – see front matter © 2012 Elsevier Inc. All rights reserved.

and successfully applied for discovery of serum and tissue markers for different types of cancers.[13,14] Various label-based detection systems using fluorescent dyes, chemiluminescent agents, radioisotopes, epitope tags, and, more recently, quantum dots and gold nanoparticles, are commonly implicated in protein microarrays for detection or amplification of signals.[15] Although the labeling strategies are used widely because of the simple instrument requirements and easy availability of reagents, the labeling procedure is laborious and time consuming and limits the number and types of analytes that can be studied simultaneously.[16] To eliminate the interference caused by the tagging, various label-free approaches, including surface plasmon resonance (SPR)-based techniques (SPR and SPR imaging [SPRi]), nanomaterial-based techniques, nanohole arrays, and interferometric assays have emerged.[17] Such label-free techniques rely on the measurement of some inherent properties of the query molecules (eg, mass and dielectric property) and allow direct, real-time detection of biomolecules in an HT manner, eliminating the requirement of any secondary reactants.

SPR is one of the most promising label-free approaches for studying molecular interactions,[18] real-time binding kinetics,[19] and surface characteristics of molecules[20](**Fig. 1**). SPR occurs when energy from the monochromatic incident light beam strikes the metal-dielectric interface at a particular SPR angle and gets transformed into electromagnetic energy leading to the generation of evanescent waves. The extent of SPR depends on many factors, including nature of the metal layer, SPR angle, incident light wavelength, and refractive index at the metal-dielectric interface etc.[21] The limit of detection of conventional SPR is in picomolar range,[22] which is still insufficient for the detection of very low abundance markers in complex biological fluids and needs to be explored further. Recent advancements in the field of SPR mainly focused on the introduction of new materials and methods for the improvement of sensitivity of the instruments.[23] To this end, a few interesting achievements have recently been made to improve the coupling of incident light to plasmons, to enhance surface plasmon excitations using different polarization methods for the incident light (such as p-polarized, s-polarized, TM waves, TE waves).[24] SPRi is another advancement to perform interaction studies in an HT manner, which is not possible by conventional SPR. The basic principle of SPRi is similar to that of SPR, but intensity of the incident light as well as wavelength remains constant, and the reflected light is measured at an optimum reflectance angle coming from the metal interface, and the whole array can be captured by coupled charge device (CCD) camera for HT studies.[25] SPR-based biosensors capable of detecting very minute amounts of target analytes with high selectivity have attracted considerable attention for discovery of cancer biomarkers. In this article, we discuss the applications of SPR-based biosensing approaches for biomarker discovery in different cancers. Existing challenges and major technologic advancements of SPR have also been discussed in the light of clinical applications.

## APPLICATION OF SPR-BASED SENSING TECHNIQUES IN CANCER BIOMARKER DETECTION

Label-free approaches are capable of rapid and real-time detection of target proteins. Among different types of emerging label-free detection techniques, SPR and SPRi are considered as the most potential alternative to label-based detection techniques because they offer nearly comparable sensitivity (picomolar level) to single-color and dual-color labeling approaches. SPR-based sensing approaches have gained popularity in a wide range of applications due to their accuracy, sensitivity, and real-time and label-free detection capability. Coupling of different signal amplifiers, such as

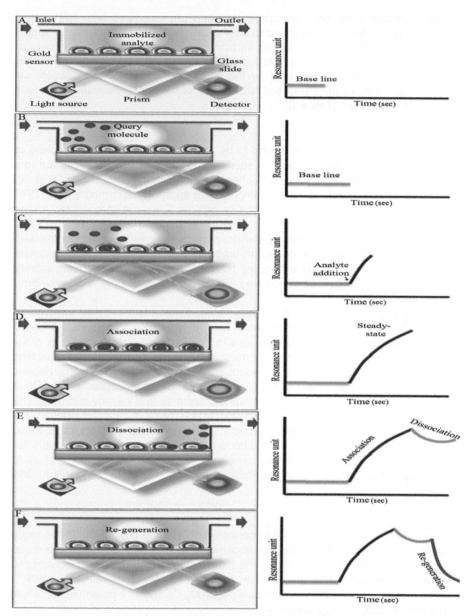

**Fig. 1.** Stepwise analysis of biomolecular interaction using SPR sensor. SPR is a surface-sensitive technique with ability to monitor the interaction between different types of molecules by measuring the change in the reflectance angle arising from the metal–liquid interface. Overall SPR setup includes the incident light source, sensor gold surface, and the detector to capture the reflected light. The interaction between the molecules is detected by plotting the sensorgram (*A–F*). The ligand molecules are immobilized on an activated gold sensor chip via thiol interactions. Query molecule in buffer is flowed through the flow cell to study the interaction in a real-time manner as well as binding kinetics by measuring the association and dissociation constants.

enzyme, quantum dots, gold nanoparticles, and microspheres with SPR-based approaches have effectively improved the sensitivity limit from micromolar to femto-molar range.[15,17] SPRi is an advanced version of SPR, in which large numbers of molecular interactions can be studied simultaneously by illuminating the whole surface and capturing reflected light by the CCD camera.[26,27] In this section, we discuss the applications of SPR-based techniques for biomarker detection in various types of human cancers (**Table 1**).

### Oral Cancer

SPR-based techniques have been found to be applicable for real-time monitoring of the levels of cancer-related proteins in saliva samples.[28] In this study, the authors have designed an immunoassay for detection and quantitation of interleukin-8 (IL-8), which plays a crucial role in oral cancer, in pM range applying the combination of SPR and microfluidics. The monoclonal antibodies against IL-8 were immobilized on the gold sensor surface and modified with carboxymethyl dextran via amine groups. The saliva samples from cancer patients and healthy subjects were passed through the flow cell, and the detection was carried out by a sandwich method applying two monoclonal IL-8 antibodies having different epitope binding affinity for IL-8. The detection limit obtained was 30 and 86 pM in healthy and carcinoma patients, respectively.

The level of cyclooxygenase 2 (COX-2), a lipid metabolic enzyme involved in conversion of essential lipid arachidonic acid to the prostaglandins, increased radically in oral precancerous lesions, oral squamous cell carcinoma, and other malignant cancers.[29] Although the exact mechanism is not clear, it is suggested that COX-2 increases malignancy by the production of prostaglandins. Recently, Kapoor and colleagues[30] have reported the application of SPR for the measurement of COX-2 levels in diluted plasma samples of oral cancer patients and healthy subjects. The authors have reported around 3 times increase in plasma COX-2 level during the late stage of oral cancer and metastatic cervical lymph node. Elevated levels of these candidate proteins under diseased conditions can be utilized as good indicators for early detection as well as monitoring cancer progression, but specificity of such disease surrogates needs to be established before developing any diagnostic approach.

### Pancreatic Cancer

Pancreatic cancer is the fourth leading cancer in developing countries. On the basis of site of tumor growth, pancreatic cancer can be classified into two types, the major adenocarcinoma, which mostly affects the digestive juice synthesizing duct, and the minor endocrine pancreatic cancer, which affects the hormone-releasing cells.[31] Activated leukocyte cell adhesive molecule (ALCAM), CD166, is a potential biomarker for pancreatic cancer progression. Although enzyme-linked immunosorbent assay (ELISA) kits for ALCAM are commercially available, the time requirements, high labelling costs, and paucity of multiplexing capability lead to the requirement of sensitive and cost-effective alternative detection approaches. To this end, SPR provides an attractive option. Recently, Vaisocherová and coworkers compared the efficiency of SPR-based detection assay and conventional ELISA techniques for detection of ALCAM levels in buffer as well as in serum samples of healthy subjects and pancreatic cancer patients.[32] Similar detection limit (~0.5 ng/mL) was obtained for both of the detection approaches for the target biomarker.

More recently, SPRi has been applied for detection of two model cancer biomark-ers; human chorionic gonadotropin and ALCAM in tris-EDTA-NaCl (TENα) buffer and blood plasma.[33] Authors have adopted a DNA-based functionalization approach using antibodies conjugated with oligonucleotides via thiolated groups (**Fig. 2**). Before passing the samples through the flow cell, the array surface was blocked with bovine serum albumin to improve the sensitivity and reduce the background noise. Detection limit at nanogram per milliliter level was obtained for both the target proteins.[33] Such successful studies confirm the potential of SPR-based sensing approaches for the direct detection of biomarkers for pancreatic and other types of cancers in different biological fluids (see **Table 1**).

*Prostate Cancer*
***

Prostate cancer Is the third most dangerous cancer affecting the prostate glands, occurring mostly in men older than 50 years. Blood level of prostate-specific antigen (PSA) is a good indicator for the detection of prostate cancer. Diagnosis of prostate cancer at an early stage requires highly sensitive diagnostic tests, which can detect the ultra-low levels of PSA in blood samples. Choi and colleagues[34] have designed an SPR-based immunosensor with a gold surface coated with PSA monoclonal antibodies (mAbs) and gold nanoparticle–conjugated antibody complex, where PSA antigen was specifically bound to the mAbs coated on gold surface.[34] Sensitivity of the technique was enhanced effectively (down to 300 fM of the target molecule) by tagging the antigen with a complex having gold nanoparticle–conjugated PSA polyclonal Abs (**Fig. 3**). Validation of shift in SPR angle was carried out by SPR spectroscopy to test whether the shift in angle is caused by the gold nanoparticles alone or the gold nanoparticle–conjugated antibody complex by measuring the absorbance at $A_{525}$ and $A_{280}$, respectively.

Another advanced form of SPR technology for HT screening of disease biomarkers is localized SPR (LSPR), where noble metal nanoparticles are used to release electron by light induction. Interesting properties of noble metals, such as increased electromagnetic field at the surface of the nanoparticle and highly sensitive spectrum to the local environmental refractive index at the nanoparticles surface, are being utilized to enhance the efficacy and sensitivity of the approach. LSPR immunoassay is one of the highly sensitive detection methods for cancer biomarkers, and a proof-of-concept study was performed using PSA. David and coworkers developed an LSPR system with a monolayer of silver nanoparticles coated with octanethiol and mercaptoundecanoic acid, above which PSA antibodies were immobilized with different concentrations for selective detection of the target (**Fig. 4**).[35] Very recently, Krishnan and coworkers[36] showed the detection of ultralow concentration of PSA using SPR-based immunosensing. Such ultrasensitive detection platforms will be very useful for cancer diagnostics once the efficiency, sensitivity, and specificity of the technology remains unaffected during analysis of real biological samples.

PSA is considered a well-known marker for prostate cancer diagnosis, but increased levels of PSA are also observed in other diseases, like benign prostates disease (BPD). Therefore, accurate diagnosis requires the identification of multiple biomarkers with high specificity. Recently, some acute-phase proteins have been reported to exhibit enhanced expression levels in different types of cancers. Among the interesting candidates, haptoglobin has attained considerable importance. In prostate cancer, increased glycosylation of haptoglobin is observed, and measurement of the glycosylated protein is useful to monitor the progression of the disease.[37] Kazuno and colleagues[38] designed a sequential SPR with immobilized antihaptoglobin polyclonal antibodies on the sensor chip, and the amount of glycosylation of haptoglobin was measured by taking the resonance unit of lectin to haptoglobin. Coupling of SPRi technology with high molecular weight biotin-streptavidin probes

**Table 1**
Cancer biomarker discovery by SPR

| Study | Type of Cancer | Findings | Limit of Detection | Principle |
|---|---|---|---|---|
| Carrascosa et al[48] | Breast cancer | BRCA1 mutations | 50 nM | DNA functionalization through verticaland lateral nucleotide spacers on SPR sensor |
| Chang et al[49] | | CA-15.3 | 0.025 U/mL | Analytes are coated on Au/ZnO nanocomposite for SPR sensor surface |
| Myung et al[50] | | CD24 | NA* | E-selectin functionalized SPR having 2 channels, ie, for reference as well as sample |
| Singh et al[71] | | Lipoxygenase-12 (LOX-12) | $8.9 \times 10^{-2}$ ng/mL | Human IgG LOX antibodies are immobilized on sensor chip, through flow cell, different concentrations of purified proteins, and sera passed separately |
| Yang et al[28] | Oral cancer | IL-8 | 250 pM | SPR with microfluidic channel |
| Kapoor et al[30] | | COX-2 | NA* | Anti-COX antibody functionalized SPR sensor |
| Vaisocherová et al[32] | Pancreatic cancer | ALCAM | 0.5–1 ng/mL | Four channel SPR with anti-ALCAM and anti-salmonella antibody |
| Piliarik et al[33] | | ALCAM & hCG | 45 & 100 ng | SPR imaging with functionalized antibody biosensor chip via oligonucleotide linker |
| Choi et al[34] | Prostate cancer | PSA | 300 fM | SPR immunosensor with gold nanoparticle antibody complex for detection |
| Malic et al[25] | | PSA-ACT complex | 100 pg/mL | SPR imaging signal enhancement with quantum dots |
| Jang et al[72] | | PSA-ACT complex | 4 ng/mL | Few mode fiber surface plasmon resonance functionalized PSA-Act complex and detection by sandwich method with pPSA complex |
| Krishnan et al[36] | | PSA | 300 aM | SPR with supramagnetic labels for signal enhancement |
| Cao et al[73] | | PSA-ACT complex | 10.2 ng/mL | SPR immunosensor chip functionalized using a mixture of EG6-COOH and EG3-OH |
| David et al[35] | | PSA | 10 nM | Localized SPR bionanosensor |
| Kazuno et al[38] | | Haptoglobin | 10 ng | Sequential SPR having immobilized anti-haptoglobin antibodies, and detection of glycosylation is carried out by passing various lectins |

| Reference | Cancer type | Biomarker | Detection limit | Method |
| --- | --- | --- | --- | --- |
| Su et al[39] | Colorectal cancer | CEA | 25 ng/mL | SPR biosensor having immobilized anti-CEA antibody via Protein-G or Protein-A |
| Ladd et al[40] | | CEA autoantibody | 125 ng/mL | SPR immunosensor with HRP conjugated antibody for signal enhancement |
| Li et al[42] | | VEGF protein | Pico molar | RNA aptamer coupled SPR technology |
| Ladd et al[41] | | ALCAM/CD 166 &transgelin-2 | 6 & 3 ng/mL | SPR imaging with polarizer to enhance the signal sensitivity |
| Teramura & Iwata[43] | Hepatocellular carcinoma | AFP | 700 ng/mL | Sandwich detection system on SPR sensor |
| Fang et al[45] | Gastric cancer | MG-7 | NA* | SPR sensor platform |
| Law et al[22] | Other cancers | TNF-$\alpha$ | 0.03 pM | SPR immunoassay with gold nanorod coupled detection antibody |
| Suwansa-ard et al[74] | | CA 125 | 0.1 U/mL | SPR immunosensor with anti-CA 125 immobilization |

aNot available.

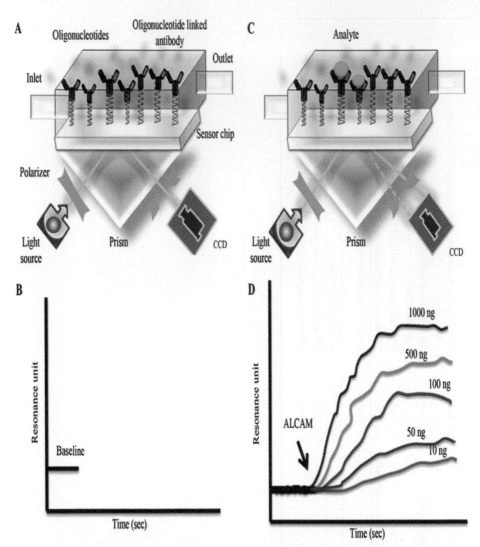

**Fig. 2.** Coupling of SPR with antibody microarray. (*A*) SPR setup includes 2 polarizers; one after the incident light source and the second just before the detector. To immobilize the antibodies on the sensor chip, the chip is functionalized with oligonucleotides through thiol groups, followed by the immobilization of the antibodies conjugated with oligonucleotides through the hybridization between the complimentary strands.[33] (*B*) The sensorgram indicates the baseline before the addition of any query molecule. (*C*) Potential interacting partners are passed through the flow cell for interaction analysis. (*D*) The sensorgram indicates the response of the antibody microarray sensor to the different concentrations of the target molecules. Gradual enhancement of the shift in reflectance angle with the increase in the concentration of the target molecules indicates a direct interaction.

and various nanoparticle conjugates, like gold nanoparticles and silicon gold nanorods, can significantly improve the sensitivity. Malic and coworkers[25] have used quantum dots (QD)-conjugated probes to detect the cDNA and PSA-alpha 1-antichymotrypsin (ACT) complex. In this assay, the investigators designed a

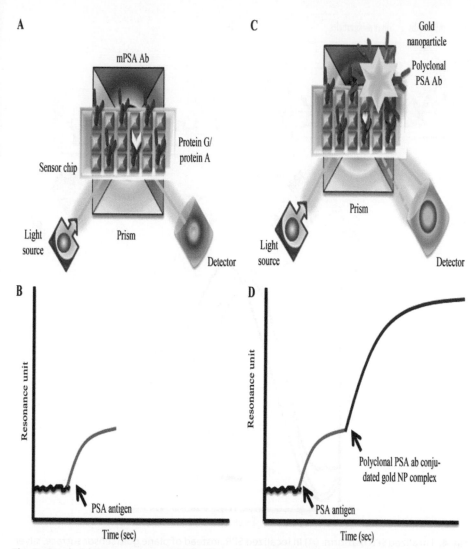

**Fig. 3.** Sandwich immunoassay SPR platform for detection of target antigen (PSA as a model candidate). (*A*) Gold sensor chip functionalized with recombinant protein G via thiol groups, above which PSA monoclonal antibodies were coated for interaction studies.[34] (*B*) The sensorgram indicates the binding of the target antigen with immobilized antibodies. However, the change in SPR angle is insufficient to monitor such interactions in complex clinical samples. (*C*) The interaction can be studied either by direct measurement of the SPR angle or by using a sandwich immunoassay approach using gold nanoparticle conjugated with PSA polyclonal antibody complex. (*D*) Application of gold nanoparticle-antibody complex as signal amplifier significantly improved the sensitivity level.

functionalized gold surface with calixcrown-capture antibody (cAb) and probed with PSA-ACT complex. The first stage of signal amplification was carried out by biotinylated detection antibody (dAb) followed by further amplification by streptavidin-conjugated QDs (**Fig. 5**). This sandwich detection system with QDs allowed

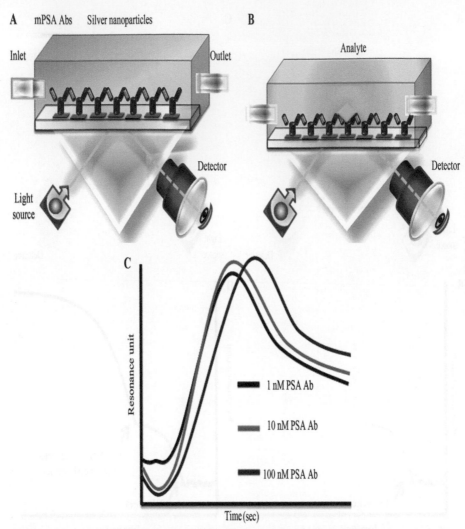

**Fig. 4.** Localized SPR platform. (*A*) In localized SPR, instead of plane gold sensor surface, silver nanoparticles coated SAM layer was used. Treatment of silver nanoparticles with octanethiol and mercaptoundecanoic acid formed the SAM layer and above it the monoclonal PSA antibodies were immobilized for interaction analysis.[35] (*B*) Different concentrations of the target antigen (PSA) were passed through the flow cell. (*C*) The sensorgram represents the enhancement in SPR angle with the increase in the concentration of the target analyte.

the differentiation of PSA-ACT levels between the control subjects and patients at very low levels, which was not possible to measure by SPRi alone.

### Colorectal Cancer

Carcinoembryonic antigen (CEA) is a cell membrane glycoprotein involved in cell adhesion and considered a detection surrogate for colorectal, breast, and other cancers. The normal levels of CEA in serum of healthy individuals and smokers are 2.5 ng/mL and

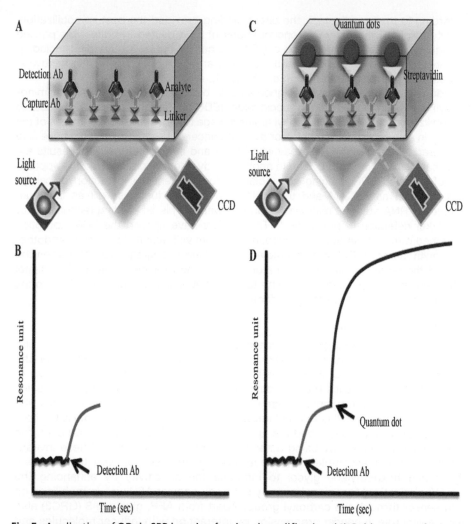

**Fig. 5.** Application of QDs in SPR imaging for signal amplification. (*A*) Gold sensor surface was functionalized with linkers to immobilize the capture antibodies against PSA-ACT complex.[25] (*B*) SPR angle shift was less when the detection was carried out with detection antibody alone. (*C*) Analytes having PSA-ACT complex were passed through the surface to monitor the levels of PSA-ACT antigen. Detection was carried out at 2 levels, first with biotin-conjugated PSA-ACT antibody, and the second level detection was performed by streptavidin-conjugated QDs. (*D*) Sensorgram indicates that streptavidin-conjugated QDs improved the limit of detection to picograms range.

5 ng/mL, respectively, whereas the level is increased up to 100 ng/mL in tumor conditions. Su and colleagues[39] have tested various sensor surface modifications and binding chemistry to achieve improved sensitivity for the target antigens using SPR technology. In SPR, antibodies are generally immobilized on the sensor chip by direct binding to the surface or by using capture molecule through covalent interaction. In this study, the authors used 4 different methods, including direct binding and binding through protein A, protein G, and antimouse IgG polyclonal antibodies against CEA.

According to the investigators, the direct binding provided the best immobilization. Analyte solution with different concentrations of CEA diluted in buffer was passed through the flow cell, and detection of CEA was carried out by 3 antibodies, including capture antibody RDI, anti-CEA antibody, and anti-CEA antibody for the sandwich detection with an limit of detection of 25 ng/mL.

Ladd and coworkers[40] have designed an SPR biosensor with ethyl(dimethylamino-propyl) carbodiimide/N-Hydroxysuccinimide (EDC/NHS) functionalized surface to immobilize the CEA through carboxyl amine linkage to detect the concentration of the antigen in sera samples from colon or ovarian cancer patients. The authors have also compared the sandwich SPR assay with ELISA and concluded that SPR results are significantly matching with ELISA. In another study, the authors showed the application of modified SPR imaging with polarizer for the sensitive detection of cancer markers such as ALCAM and transgelin-2 in purified form as well as in serum samples.[41] RNA aptamer microarray coupled with SPR is an exciting technology for biomarker detection in pM range.[42] The authors have applied the SPRi approach combined with an RNA aptamer microarray system with affinity to vascular endothe-lial growth factor (VEGF), a signal molecule involved in angiogenesis, to screen the level of the target marker in rheumatoid arthritis and cancer patients. The signal enhancement was achieved by adding tetramethylbenzidine substrate, which forms insoluble complex on the sensor surface (**Fig. 6**).

### Hepatocellular Carcinoma

Hepatocellular carcinoma (HCC) is one of the major cancers affecting the liver and causing millions of deaths annually. In HCC, the survival rate is rare after the diagnosis, and the rate of mortality is increasing every year. The principle cause of HCC is 2 viruses, hepatitis B and hepatitis C virus, along with few minor factors like aflatoxins, alcohol consumption, hemochromatosis, tyrosinemia, and Wilson's dis-ease. A-fetoprotein (AFP) is the well known marker for the diagnosis of HCC.There are reports that have described the applications of SPR technology to detect the AFP in nanogram level by using a sandwich detection method.[43] These investi-gators used self assembled monolayer-coated gold sensor with tetraethylene glycol and hexaethylene glycol to increase the sensitivity by enhancing the signal/noise ratio. Monoclonal primary antibody against AFP was immobilized on gold sensor through the carboxyl group. Apart from AFP, glypican 3 (GPC3) also plays a vital role in cancer progression by interaction with inducer molecules and is considered a potential biomarker for HCC. GPC3 is a heparin sulfate proteogly-can with integral membrane protein and varying sugar moieties. Cho and colleagues[44] have applied the SPR-based sensing approach for studying the interaction between GPC3 and glucose transporter 1 (GLUT1) and its effect on glucose transport activity in HCC cells. The results obtained from SPR analysis and other immunoassay-based confirmatory tests, including immunoprecipitation (IP)-western blot, established that GLUT1 binds to C-terminal cell surface-attached form of GPC3 with an equilibrium dissociation constant of 1.61 nM, resulting a reduction in the glucose transport activity in HCC.

### Gastric Cancer

Gastric cancer is the second most dreadful malignant cancer and lacks any well-established early stage diagnosis assays. MG-7 Abs are considered as the potential biomarkers for gastric cancer diagnosis.[45] Investigators have used gold sensor surface modified with 3-merceptopropionic acid to immobilize the MG-7 Ab. SPR sensor was used to detect MG-7 Ag in cell lysate from MKN45 gastric cell lines

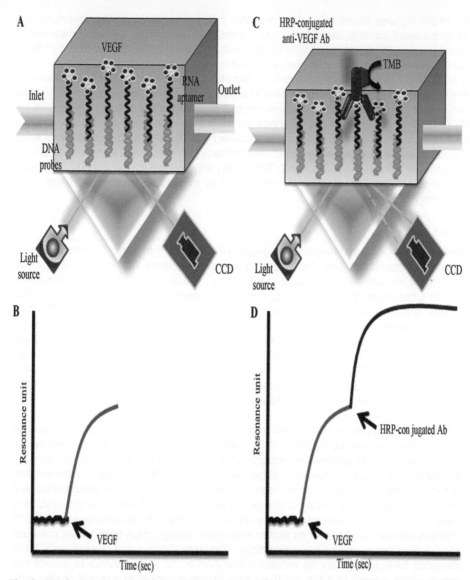

**Fig. 6.** SPR imaging using RNA aptamer. (*A*) RNA aptamer microarray fabrication on the SPR imaging platform involves 2 steps; initially the sensor surface was fabricated with ssDNA probes via 3'-OH group and free 5'-phophate group. Later, ssRNA probes having 3'-OH group were added to the chip along with RNA ligase, so that the ligase can make the phosphodiester bond between ssDNA and ssRNA to fabricate the RNA aptamers.[42] (*B*) The query molecule exhibited lower shifts in resonance angle. (*C*) The whole setup was used to monitor the VEGF levels in serum. (*D*) Signal enhancement was carried out by horseradish peroxidase-conjugated anti-VEGF antibody and TMB substrate.

and sera from gastric cancer patients and healthy controls. In every case, the shift in wavelength was measured by passing the cell lysates and sera samples in different platforms using the same methodology. The net shift in wavelength was measured by subtracting the baseline with only phosphate buffer saline. The shift in the wavelength for MG-7 Ag was found to be 11.9 nm with cell lysate, 10.9 nm with serum from a gastric cancer patient, and 5.4 nm with control sera. Recently, Liu and coworkers[46] designed an SPR platform by immobilizing live cells on the gold sensor chip by taking BGC823 cell lines as a model. Live cells having membrane receptors or proteins were able to bind on poly-L-lysine–coated sensor chip and formed a flattened layer so that the maximum portion of receptor was in close proximity to the sensor surface. The SPR setup also contained temperature control to maintain the cells in living condition, CCD camera to capture the changes in morphology of cell periodically, and a reference sensor surface having immobilized fixed cells.[46] Immunofluorescence detection of the SPR signal helped to discriminate between the live and dead cells on the basis of the lifetime of the signal. This study showed the ability of SPR biosensors for detection of mismatch sequences related to inherited breast cancer, with high specificity and sensitivity.

### Breast Cancer

Breast cancer is a heterogeneous group of cancers that form in breast tissue, commonly the ducts and lobules, and occurs in many forms such as ductal carcinoma *in situ* or intraductal carcinoma, which is an invasive carcinoma affecting the lining of the milk ducts, and lobular carcinoma *in situ*.[47] In spite of the notable advancement in cancer diagnostics over the last decade, the effective screening and prevention methods remain to be explored further. The priority of current medical research is identification of disease biomarkers that can help detect and treat the disease(s) at early stages and application of those identified targets in clinics. Detection of cancer-causing DNA mutations by the traditional molecular biology techniques is expensive, tedious, and time consuming. SPR is an emerging alternative approach to monitor the DNA interaction studies with high sensitivity and specificity.[48]

Gold-coated glass slides are used widely as a sensor in conventional SPR because of their ability to excite electrons and simple binding by thiol groups. However, because of the poor adherence property of glass, chromium (Cr) nanomaterials are applied to enhance the adherence of gold to the glass slide. Although Cr nanomaterials are used commonly in conventional methods, Cr is not an ideal metal because it changes the optical properties of the gold film by metal diffusion. To this end, zinc oxide (ZnO) is an attractive semiconductor nanomaterial for biosensors as well as in chemical sensors because of its higher excitation energy, high transparent conductance, low resistance, and high specificity. Recently, Chang and colleagues[49] have advanced SPR technology by replacing the Au/Cr film with Au/ZnO to detect the carbohydrate antigen 15.3 (CA-15.3) markers in breast cancer as a model protein with a detection limit of 0.025 U/mL. Cancer metastasis is promoted by interacting rolling cancer cells with specific receptors to the endothelium via selectin glycol-proteins. Among the selectins, E-selectin is the major protein involved in metastasis in various cancers by adhering to wide range of ligands. Hong and coworkers[50] have demonstrated that MCF-7 cells exhibit rolling response on immobilized E-selectin and hypothesized that CD24 is the ligand responsible for invasion and metastasis. To test the hypothesis, the authors used an SPR-based sensing approach, where E-selectin was immobilized on SPR gold sensor surface and the recombinant CD24 and a positive control, sLeX, were passed through the flow cell. The direct interaction between CD24 and E-selectin was detected by monitoring the sensorgram, and the association and dissociation rate constant parameters suggested that CD24 binds to E-selectin more strongly than the positive control (**Fig. 7**).

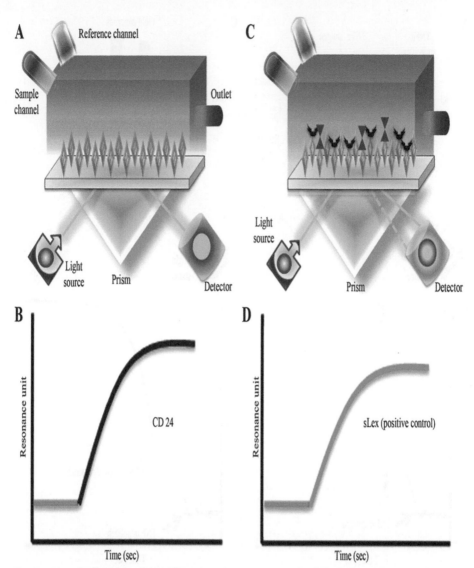

**Fig. 7.** SPR platform for identification of CD24 partners. (*A*) Rolling of tumor cells on E-selectin surface leads to metastasis, but the inducer responsible for rolling is not known. E-selectins were immobilized on the functionalized gold sensor chip. (*C*) CD24, which was hypothesized as an inducer and sLex, which is a positive control, was passed through the flow cell with 2 channels, one for CD24 and the other as a reference channel to study the interaction as well as binding kinetics.[50] (*B, D*) The sensorgram indicates that both CD24 and sLex have shown interaction. CD24 exhibited stronger interaction than the positive control.

### Other Cancers

Tumor necrosis factor alpha (TNF-$\alpha$) is a cytokine involved in acute phase inflammation and considered a potential diagnostic biomarker in many cancers. Conventional methods are not sensitive enough to monitor the levels of TNF-$\alpha$ in serum. Recently,

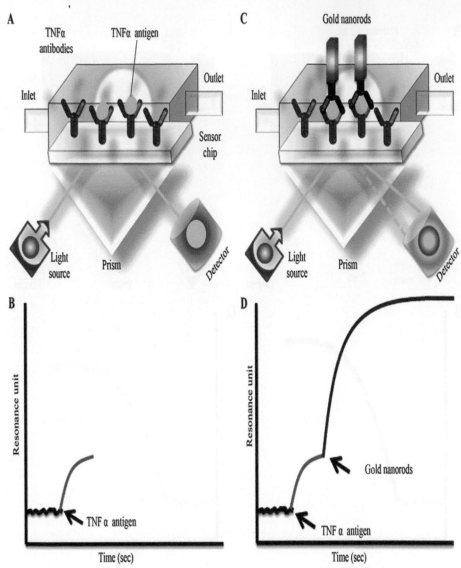

**Fig. 8.** Application of gold nanorods in SPR sensor. (*A*) TNF-α antibodies were immobilized on a CM-5 gold sensor chip, which was activated with EDC and NHC.[22]\(*B*) The sensorgram when only TNF-α was bound to the antibody on sensor chip. (*C*) The detection antibodies were functionalized on gold nanorod by incubating for 30 minutes; dAb-gold nanorods were separated by centrifugation. Solution containing TNF-α was passed through the flow cell followed by the passing of dAb-gold nanorods.(*D*) The sensorgram exhibited the higher sensitivity with gold nanorods–conjugated detection antibody.

Law and colleagues[22] have introduced SPR immunoassay with gold nanorod (GNR)-coupled antibodies to detect the target cytokine at pM (0.03 pM) level. Captured antibodies against TNF-α were immobilized on the CM-5 gold sensor chip after activating with EDC and NHS, and TNF-α was passed through the flow cell (**Fig. 8**).

The sensitivity of the detection method was enhanced significantly because of the use of GNR-conjugated antibodies. These successful studies indicate that the diagnostic applications of SPR biosensors are promising and can be translated into real clinical applications once such sensing methods retain their efficiency during the *in vivo* assays with an affordable overall assay cost.

## SCREENING OF INHIBITORS OF TUMOR TARGETS BY SPR

Beside biomarker detection, SPR is also an attractive approach for real-time analysis of different biomolecular interactions, including protein-protein, protein-DNA, DNA-DNA, and protein-drug along with interaction kinetics. Multiple studies have confirmed the efficiency of this label-free HT technology for studying inhibitors against potential cancer targets and screening novel inhibitors for targeting tumors.[51–53] In this section we discuss a few interesting studies that have used SPR technology for real-time interaction analysis as well as screening of different inhibitors (**Table 2**).

Cancer metastasis occurs through blood vessels and the lymphatic system. CCL21, the most important chemokine for lymphatic invasion associated to cancer, can be used as a potential target for cancer treatment by blocking its interaction with the receptor CCL7. Lanati and coworkers[51] have carried out a yeast 2-hybrid screening of the natural high endothelial venule c-DNA library to synthesize the human zinc finger binding motif with an ability to bind with CCL21 to stop its function both *in vitro* and *in vivo*. To confirm the interaction, purified THAP1 and chemotrap-1 were immobilized on gold sensor chip, and CCL21 was passed in a fixed concentration through the flow cell. The association and dissociation constants for the interaction were studied by passing the different concentrations of purified CCL21. The complex of urokinase-receptor (uPAR) and its partner molecule, urokinase-type activating plasminogen (uPA), bound to the cell surface receptors, such as tyrosine kinase, integrins, GPCRs leading to the progression of tumor, proliferation, angiogenesis, and metastasis. Antibiotics, antibodies or any small molecules that can inhibit the activity of uPA by hampering the activation of plasminogen and prevents the interaction between uPAR-uPA are very attractive from a therapeutic point of view. Recently, Khanna and coworkers[52] screened 10,000 small molecules to check their ability to inhibit the uPAR-uPA interaction by using docking and molecular dynamic simulations. Validation of the small molecule inhibitors for protein-protein interactions was executed by using SPR assay. In this experimental setup, the amino terminal uPA was immobilized on a CM-dextran gold surface, and the uPAR protein was passed through the flow cell with different concentrations of IPR-763 and IPR-803 to detect the $IC_{50}$ for the inhibition.

The overexpression of aurora kinases is a common phenomenon in different types of cancers because they are involved in mitosis and regulate cell divisions. Targeting aurora kinases by blocking the downstream partners or ATP binding sites by small molecules is an interesting approach for cancer therapy. To this end, selective inhibition of the functions of aurora kinases is possible by blocking the downstream partners or ATP binding sites by applying small molecules. Lang and colleagues[54] have carried out an HT screening of 70,000 small molecules against aurora B and selected 80 compounds showing potential activity with IC50 is less than 10 $\mu M$. Validation of direct interaction between Aurora B and one of the selected candidates, 3-hydroxyflavon, was carried out by SPR.[54] Pololike kinase 1 is another important kinase involved in mitotic cell progression and exhibits overexpression in many cancers as well as cancer cell lines. Binding of the small molecules to the ATP binding pocket or polo box domain pocket of pololike kinase 1 can inhibit its catalytic activity. Akt and C-Src are also involved in cell cycle progression, metabolism, survival, and

**Table 2**
Cancer inhibitory study by SPR

| Study | Type of Cancer/Cell Line | Target | Drug Used |
|---|---|---|---|
| Lanati et al[51] | Melanoma cells | CCL21 | Chemotrap -1 |
| Khanna et al[52] | MDA-MB-231 breast cancer cell lines | uPAR-uPA interaction | IPR-456 |
| Lang et al[54] | Colon, breast, gastric cancers (HeLa cell lines) | Aurora kinases | 3-hydroxyflavon |
| Li et al[55] | HeLa, A549, HGC & HCT-8/V cells | Pololike kinase 1 | Aristolactam AllIa |
| Mine et al[75] | COR-L23, MIAPaCa2 and NCI-H226 cell lines | Calmodulin and arrest cell cycle at G2 phase | CBP-501 |
| Estrada et al[53] | Prostate cancer (LNCaP and PC-3 cell lines) | Akt kinases | Tirucallic acid |
| Ma et al[56] | Breast cancer (MDA-MB-231andMDA-MB-435 cell lines) | c-Src-kinase | PH006 |
| Ma et al[76] | HMECs cell lines | Tyrosine kinase | Marine-derived oligosaccharide sulfate |
| Ahad et al[77] | BxPC-3 cells | Phosphatidylinositol 3-kinase/AKT signaling pathway | Sulfonamides |
| Lu et al[58] | Colorectal carcinoma HCT116cells | Tubulin | Curcumin |
| Basappa et al[60] | Osteosarcoma cell line LM8G7 &human ovarian cell lines, OVSAHO and SKOV-3 | VEGF, HB-EGF & TNF-α | DMBO |
| Vicari et al[78] | HUVEC cell lines | VEGF signaling | VEGF-P3 cyclic peptide |
| Matthews et al[79] | Breast cancer cell lines | ErbB | Mini RNA aptamer |
| Macias et al[65] | BL21 (purified protein) | Grp78 | VER-155008 |
| Horibe et al[66] | BT-20, T47D, MDA-MB-231, A549, Caki-1, LNCap, OE19, MRC5 and BXPC3 cell lines | Hsp90 | TRP peptide |
| Musso et al[67] | Human ovarian carcinoma cell line IGROV-1, melanoma cell line JR8 and epithelial carcinoma cell line A431 | Hsp90 | Bulgarialactone B |

| Matthews et al[79] | LNCaP and PC-3 cell lines | Hsp90 | F-4 an novobiocin analogue |
|---|---|---|---|
| Ban et al[63] | SW620, HCT116 (p53 +/+), and HCT116 (p53 −/−) Colon cancer cell lines | NF-kB | Inflexinol |
| Chang et al[80] | Lung cancer & colorectal cancer (purified protein from BL21) | PGE2 syntheses | PGE0001 (Aminothiazole scaffold) |
| Chen et al[81] | MDA-MB-468 & HT-29 | Protein tyrosine phosphatase (PTP) Shp2 | SPI-112 |
| Chen et al[82] | HT-29 and MCF-7 cell lines | Id1 (inhibitor of DNA-binding protein) | MyoD peptide fragments |
| Liu et al[83] | Many cancers | Integrin $\alpha_v\beta_3$ | Cyclopeptide c-lys |
| Qiu et al[84] | MCF-7 cell lines | Human phosphatidylethanolamine-binding protein 4 (hPEBP4) | IOI-42 |
| Erkizan et al[85] | Ewing tumor cells | EWS-FLI1 | ESAP1 |
| Bulut et al[86] | Zebrafish, Xenopus | Ezrin | NSC305787 and NSC668394 |

growth. These kinases exhibit enhanced activity under a cancerous state and are potential targets for the development of novel anticancer drugs. SPR-based sensing platform has been found to be very effective for HT screening of large number of small molecule inhibitors against these target enzymes.[53,55,56] Such HT screening ability poses tremendous potential to provide a wealth of new information to accelerate cancer research and aid in the identification of new anticancer drugs.

Identification of small molecules or drugs having inhibitory action on enzymes that play a vital role in cancer progression and metastasis is one of the major goals for cancer research. Curcumin, a dietary pigment obtained from plants, have multiple targets in cancer cells, and, according to the recent studies, it has the ability to damage the DNA leading to the activation of 2 kinases, ataxia-telangiectasia-mutated (ATM) and Rad3-related (ATR), which have inhibitory effects on the cell cycle progression.[57] Recently, Lu and coworkers[58] have shown that tubulin is the major target for curcumin in colorectal carcinoma cell lines and applied SPR sensor chip to study the interaction and kinetics between purified tubulin and curcumin.[58] Heparin sulfate (HS), a polysaccharide involved in signal transduction across the cell membrane in various tumors in response to various growth factors such as VGEF, fibroblast growth factor (FGF), heparin-binding epidermal growth factor–like growth factor (HB-EGF), plays a vital role in metastasis, cell invasion, proliferation, and angiogenesis by disturbing the extracellular HS matrix and releasing growth factors.[59] Heterocyclic synthetic compounds, such as oxazines, having the ability to mimic the function of HS, are interesting candidates for cancer therapy. 2-(2,6-difluorophenyl)-5-(4-methoxy-phenyl)-1-oxa-3-azaspiro[5.5]undecane (DMBO) is one of the pyranoside oxazines that can block the function of various growth factors as well as heparin. Basappa and colleagues[60] have conducted a SPR-based assay to screen the potential small molecules that can mimic the HS by immobilizing 69 pyranosides including DMBO. The SPR analysis found significant interaction between DMBO with VEGF, TNF-$\alpha$, and HB-EGF. The authors have also introduced different substitutions on the oxazine nucleus of DMBO and established that the 2,6 difluorophenyl group is necessary for interaction with VEGF, TNF-$\alpha$, and HB-EGF but not with other growth factors (**Fig. 9**). Nuclear factor-kB (NF-kB) is an antiapoptotic transcription factor that enhances the cancer cell proliferation as well as survival rate by inhibiting the apoptotic mechanisms.[61] Many synthetic and natural products such as aspirin, ibuprofen, and various terpenoids have been tested to establish their inhibitory action on NF-kB activity.[62] Recently, Ban and colleagues[63] examined the interaction between NF-kB and inflexinol, a terpenoid from natural plant extract, using SPR. The SPR-based HT screening approach has been used successfully to screen various interesting candidate molecules with the potential to block the function of important cellular enzymes/proteins, such as ErbB, glucose-regulated protein (GRP78), HSP70, and prostaglandin E2 that play vital roles in cell division, cancer proliferation, and angiogenesis (see **Table 2**).[49,64–67] SPR-based biosensing for identification of novel target inhibitors or drug molecules from large numbers of potential candidates is very promising for cancer therapeutics. However, *in vivo* examination of the interactions is required to evaluate the actual anticancer properties of the identified molecules under real physiological conditions before perusing any clinical implication.

## CONCLUSIONS

Over the last two decades, various technological advancements have been introduced to improve the sensitivity and throughput of the SPR-based sensing approaches, and a large number of studies have used SPR for targeted discovery of potential biomarkers for different types of cancers. With introduction of unique

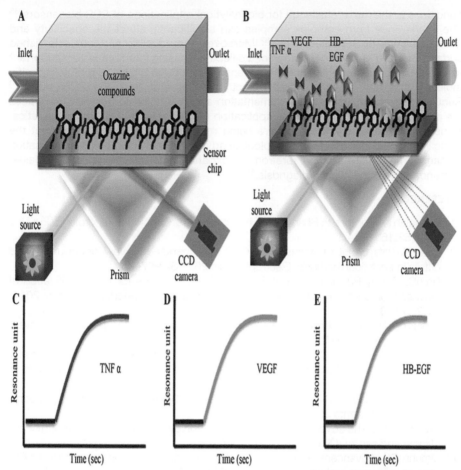

**Fig. 9.** SPRi for screening of cancer inhibitors. (*A*) Screening of small oxazine molecules, which mimics the growth factors using SPRi. Oxazine molecules were immobilized on the activated gold sensor chip through the linker molecules.[60](*B*) Different growth factors such as TNF-$\alpha$, VEGF, and HB-EGF were passed through the flow cell. (*C, D, E*) The enhanced signal intensity of DMBO was observed with TNF-$\alpha$, VEGF, and HB-EGF, and the sensorgram indicates the shift on SPR angle for all the 3 growth factors.

surface chemistry, novel materials, and advanced substrate designs, SPR-based sensing platform is evolving rapidly, and the scopes of this emerging platform have risen spectacularly in the past few years.[68] The magnitude of application of this label-free sensing approach testifies its great potential for detection of disease-specific markers and HT screening of prospective small molecules with inhibitory actions on cancer inducing enzymes, proteins, and regulators. Furthermore, combination of SPR with different technological approaches has developed extremely efficient combined techniques, such as SPRMS, electrochemical SPR and surface plasmon fluorescence spectroscopy with multidimensional applications.[69] However, at the same time, it must also be noted that despite all their promises, SPR-based approaches are still not very close from the direct large-scale clinical applications. Obtaining high sensitivity in complex biological samples under real physiological conditions is the major challenge for bioanalytical applications of SPR biosensors.[33] The interference from complex samples can significantly affect the specificity and detection limits of SPR biosensors.[32] Moreover, reproducible and well-established surface chemistry for the generation of a selective sensing interface is very important for the development of efficient SPR biosensors to reduce the binding of nonspecific moieties that can alter the local refractive index and thus the SPR signal.[70] Requirement of sophisticated instrumentation and restriction to gold/silver surfaces are also existing hindrances for the application of SPR in routine clinical diagnostics. Nonetheless, considerable efforts are being made continuously to circumvent the basic limitations, and different technological advancements, including the implication of nanoparticles, are coming forefront to expand the applications of SPR-based immunoassay to the clinical diagnosis.[16]

## REFERENCES

1. Bensalah K, Montorsi F, Shariat SF. Challenges of cancer biomarker profiling. Eur Urol 2007;52:1601–9.
2. Issaq HJ, Waybright TJ, Veenstra TD. Cancer biomarker discovery: opportunities and pitfalls in analytical methods. Electrophoresis 2011;32:967–75.
3. Ray S, Reddy PJ, Jain R. et al. Proteomic technologies for the identification of disease biomarkers in serum: advances and challenges ahead. Proteomics 2011; 11:2139–61.
4. Kijanka G, Murphy D. Protein arrays as tools for serum autoantibody marker discovery in cancer. J Proteomics 2009;72:936–44.
5. Drake RR, Cazare LH, Semmes OJ, et al. Serum, salivary and tissue proteomics for discovery of biomarkers for head and neck cancers. Expert Rev Mol Diagn 2005;5: 93–100.
6. Polanski M, Anderson NL. A list of candidate cancer biomarkers for targeted proteomics. Biomark Insights 2007;1:1–48.
7. Anderson NL. The clinical plasma proteome: a survey of clinical assays for proteins in plasma and serum. Clin Chem 2010;56:177–85.
8. Omenn GS. Advancement of biomarker discovery and validation through the HUPO plasma proteome project. Dis Markers 2004;20;131–4.
9. Wei BR, Hoover SB, Ross MM, et al. Serum S100A6 concentration predicts peritoneal tumor burden in mice with epithelial ovarian cancer and is associated with advanced stage in patients. PLoS One 2009;4:e7670.
10. Sun Y, Zang Z, Xu X, et al. Differential proteomics identification of HSP90 as potential serum biomarker in hepatocellular carcinoma by two-dimensional electrophores and mass spectrometry. Int J Mol Sci 2010;11:1423–33.
11. Ramirez AB, Loch CM, Zhang Y, et al. Use of a single-chain antibody library for ovarian cancer biomarker discovery. Mol Cell Proteomics 2010;9:1449–60.
12. Wei-Jun Q, Jon MJ, Tao L, et al. Advances and challenges in liquid chromatography-mass spectrometry based proteomic profiling for clinical applications. Mol Cell Proteomics 2006;5:1727–44.
13. Miller JC, Zhou H, Kwekel J, et al. Antibody microarray profiling of human prostate cancer sera: antibody screening and identification of potential biomarkers. Proteomics 2003;3:56–63.
14. Jaras K, Ressine A, Nilsson E, et al. Reverse phase versus sandwich antibody microarray, technical comparison from a clinical perspective. Anal Chem 2007;79: 5817–25.
15. Chandra H, Reddy PJ, Srivastava S. Protein microarrays and novel detection platforms. Expert Rev Proteomics 2011;8:61–79.

16. Srivastava S, LaBaer J. Nanotubes light up protein arrays. Nat Biotechnol 2008;26: 1244–6.
17. Ray S, Mehta G, Srivastava S. Label-free detection techniques for protein microarrays: prospects, merits and challenges. Proteomics 2010;10:731–48.
18. Kawamoto SA, Thompson AD, Coleska A, et al. Analysis of the interaction of BCL9 with beta-catenin and development of fluorescence polarization and surface plasmon resonance binding assays for this interaction. Biochemistry 2009;48:9534–41.
19. Jönsson U, Fägerstam L, Ivarsson B, et al. Real-time biospecific interaction analysis using surface plasmon resonance and a sensor chip technology. Biotechniques 1991;11:620–7.
20. Frasconi M, Tel-Vered R, Riskin M, et al. Surface plasmon resonance analysis of antibiotics using imprinted boronic acid-functionalized Au nanoparticle composites. Anal Chem 2010;82:2512–9.
21. Englebienne P,Hoonacker AV,Verhas M. Surface plasmon resonance: principles, methods and applications in biomedical sciences. Spectroscopy 2003;17:255–73.
22. Law WC, Yong KT, Baev A, et al. sensitivity improved surface plasmon resonance biosensor for cancer biomarker detection based on plasmonic enhancement. ACS Nano 2011;5:4858–64.
23. Halpern AR, Chen Y, Corn RM, et al. Surface plasmon resonance phase imaging measurements of patterned monolayers and DNA adsorption onto microarrays. Anal Chem 2011;83:2801–6.
24. Abbas A, Linman MJ, Cheng Q. New trends in instrumental design for surface plasmon resonance-based biosensors. Biosens Bioelectron 2011;26:1815–24.
25. Malic L, Sandros MG, Tabrizian M. Designed biointerface using near-infrared quantum dots for ultrasensitive surface plasmon resonance imaging biosensors. Anal-Chem 2011;83:5222–9.
26. Steiner G. Surface plasmon resonance imaging. Anal Bioanal Chem 2004;379: 328–31.
27. Lausted C, Hu Z, Hood L. Quantitative serum proteomics from surface plasmon resonance imaging. Mol Cell Proteomics 2008;7:2464–74.
28. Yang CY, Brooks E, Li Y, et al. Detection of picomolar levels of interleukin-8 in human saliva by SPR. Lab Chip 2005;5:1017–23.
29. McCormick DL, Phillips JM, Horn TL, et al. Overexpression of cyclooxygenase-2 in rat oral cancers and prevention of oral carcinogenesis in rats by selective and nonselective COX inhibitors. Cancer Prev Res (Phila) 2010;3:73–81.
30. Kapoor V, Singh AK, Dey S, et al. Circulating cycloxygenase-2 in patients with tobacco-related intraoral squamous cell carcinoma and evaluation of its peptide inhibitors as potential antitumor agent. J Cancer Res Clin Oncol 2010;136:1795–804.
31. Patra CR, Bhattacharya R, Mukhopadhyay D, et al. Fabrication of gold nanoparticles for targeted therapy in pancreatic cancer. Adv Drug Deliv Rev 2010;62:346–61.
32. Vaisocherová H, Faca VM, Taylor AD, et al. Comparative study of SPR and ELISA methods based on analysis of CD166/ALCAM levels in cancer and control human sera. Biosens Bioelectron 2009;24:2143–8.
33. Piliarik M, Bocková M, Homola J. Surface plasmon resonance biosensor for parallelized detection of protein biomarkers in diluted blood plasma. Biosens Bioelectron 2010;26:1656–61.
34. Choi JW, Kang DY, Jang YH, et al. Ultra-sensitive surface plasmon resonance based immunosensor for prostate-specific antigen using gold nanoparticle–antibody complex. Colloids and Surfaces A: physicochem. Eng Aspects 2008;313:655–9.
35. David N, Duyne RV, Bingham J. Localized surface plasmon resonance nanobiosensors for the detection of a prostate cancer biomarker. Nanoscape 2008;5:14–9.

36. Krishnan S, Mani V, Wasalathanthri D, et al. Attomolar detection of a cancer biomarker protein in serum by surface plasmon resonance using superparamagnetic particle labels. Angew Chem Int Ed Engl 2011;50:1175–8.
37. Nakano M, Nakagawa T, Ito T, et al. Site-specific analysis of N-glycans on haptoglobin in sera of patients with pancreatic cancer: a novel approach for the development of tumor markers. Int J Cancer 2008;122:2301–9.
38. Kazuno S, Fujimura T, Arai T, et al. Multi-sequential surface plasmon resonance analysis of haptoglobin–lectin complex in sera of patients with malignant and benign prostate diseases. Anal Biochem 2011;419:241–9.
39. Su F, Xu C, Taya M, et al. Detection of carcinoembryonic antigens using a surface plasmon resonance biosensor. Sensors 2008;8:4282–95.
40. Ladd J, Lu H, Taylor AD, et al. Direct detection of carcinoembryonic antigen autoantibodies in clinical human serum samples using a surface plasmon resonance sensor. Colloids Surf B Biointerfaces 2009;70:1–6.
41. Ladd J, Taylor AD, Piliarik M, et al. Label-free detection of cancer biomarker candidates using surface plasmon resonance imaging. Anal Bioanal Chem 2009;393:1157–63.
42. Li Y, Lee HJ, Corn RM. Detection of protein biomarkers using RNA aptamer microarrays and enzymatically amplified surface plasmon resonance imaging. Anal Chem 2007;79:1082–8.
43. Teramura Y, Iwata H. Label-free immunosensing for a-fetoprotein in human plasma using surface plasmon resonance. Anal Biochem 2007;365:201–7.
44. Cho HS, Ahn JM, Han HJ, et al. Glypican 3 binds to GLUT1 and decreases glucose transport activity in hepatocellular carcinoma cells. J Cell Biochem 2010;111:1252–9.
45. Fang X, Tie J, Xie Y, et al. Detection of gastric carcinoma-associated antigen MG7-Ag in human sera using surface plasmon resonance sensor. Cancer Epidemiol 2010;34:648–51.
46. Liu F, Zhang J, Den Y, et al. Detection of EGFR on living human gastric cancer BGC823 cells using surface plasmon resonance phase sensing. Sens Actuators B Chem 2011;153:398–403.
47. Sariego J, Zrada S, Byrd M, et al. Breast cancer in the young patient. Am J Surg 2010;76:1397–400.
48. Carrascosa LG, Calle A, Lechuga LM. Label-free detection of DNA mutations by SPR: application to the early detection of inherited breast cancer. Anal Bioanal Chem 2009;393:1173–82.
49. Chang CC, Chiu NF, Lin DS, et al. High-sensitivity detection of carbohydrate antigen 15-3 using a gold/zinc oxide thin film surface plasmon resonance-based biosensor. Anal Chem 2010;82:1207–12.
50. Myung JH, Launiere CA, Eddington DT, et al. Enhanced tumor cell isolation by a biomimetic combination of E-selectin and anti-EpCAM: implications for the effective separation of circulating tumor cells (CTCs). Langmuir 2010;26:8589–96.
51. Lanati S, Dunn DB, Roussigné M, et al. Chemotrap-1: an engineered soluble receptor that blocks chemokine-induced migration of metastatic cancer cells in vivo. Cancer Res 2010;70:8138–48.
52. Khanna M, Chelladurai B, Gavini A, et al. Targeting ovarian tumor cell adhesion mediated by tissue transglutaminase.Mol Cancer Ther 2011;10:626–36.
53. Estrada AC, Syrovets T, Pitterle K, et al. Tirucallic acids are novel pleckstrin homology domain-dependent akt inhibitors inducing apoptosis in prostate cancer cells. Mol Pharmacol 2010;77:378–87.
54. Lang Q, Zhang H, Li J, et al. 3-Hydroxyflavone inhibits endogenous Aurora B and induces growth inhibition of cancer cell line. Mol Biol Rep 2010;37:1577–83.

55. Li L, Wang X, Chen J, et al. The natural product Aristolactam AIIIa as a new ligand targeting the polo-box domain of polo-like kinase 1 potently inhibits cancer cell proliferation. Acta Pharmaco Sin 2009;30:1443–53.
56. Ma JG, Huang H, Chen SM, et al. PH006, a novel and selective Src kinase inhibitor, suppresses human breast cancer growth and metastasis in vitro and in vivo. Breast Cancer Res Treat 2011;130:85–96.
57. Yang J, Yu Y, Hamrick HE, et al. ATM, ATRandDNA-PK:initiatorsofthecellulargeno-toxicstress responses. Carcinogenesis 2003;24:1571–80.
58. Lu JJ, Cai YJ, Ding J. Curcumin induces DNA damage and caffeine-insensitive cell cycle arrest in colorectal carcinoma HCT116 cells. Mol Cell Biochem 2011;354:247–52.
59. Goldshmidt O, Zcharia E, Abramovitch R, et al. Cell surface expression and secretion of heparanase markedly promote tumor angiogenesis and metastasis. Proc Natl Acad Sci U S A 2002;99:10031–6.
60. Basappa NS, Elson P, Golshayan AR, et al. The impact of tumor burden character-istics in patients with metastatic renal cell carcinoma treated with sunitinib. Cancer 2011;117:1183–9.
61. Olivier S, Robe P, Bours V. Can NF-kappaB be a target for novel and efficient anti-cancer agents? Biochem Pharmacol 2006;72:1054–68.
62. Din FV, Dunlop MG, Stark LA. Evidence for colorectal cancer cell specificity of aspirin effects on NF kappa B signalling and apoptosis. Br J Cancer 2004;91:381–8.
63. Ban JO, Oh JH, Hwang BY, et al. Inflexinol inhibits colon cancer cell growth through inhibition of nuclear factor-κB activity via direct interaction with p50. Mol Cancer Ther 2009;8:1613–24.
64. Kim MY, Jeong S. In vitro selection of RNA aptamer and specific targeting of ErbB2 in breast cancer cells. Nucleic Acid Ther 2011;21:173–8.
65. Macias AT, Williamson DS, Allen N, et al. Adenosine-derived inhibitors of 78 kDa glucose regulated protein (Grp78) ATPase: insights into isoform selectivity. J Med Chem 2011;54:4034–41.
66. Horibe T, Kohno M, Haramoto M, et al. Designed hybrid TPR peptide targeting Hsp90 as a novel anticancer agent. J Transl Med 2011;9:1–8.
67. Musso L, Dallavalle S, Merlini L, et al. Natural and semisynthetic azaphilones as a new scaffold for Hsp90 inhibitors. Bioorg Med Chem 2010;18:6031–43.
68. Scarano S, Mascini M, Turner AP, et al. Surface plasmon resonance imaging for affinity-based biosensors. Biosens Bioelectron 2010;25:957–66.
69. Phillips KS, Cheng Q. Recent advances in surface plasmon resonance based tech-niques for bioanalysis. Anal Bioanal Chem 2007;387:1831–40.
70. Linman MJ, Abbas A, Cheng Q. Interface design and multiplexed analysis with surface plasmon resonance (SPR) spectroscopy and SPR imaging. Analyst 2010;135:2759–67.
71. Singh AK, Kant S, Parshad R, et al. Evaluation of human LOX-12 as a serum marker for breast cancer. Biochem Biophys Res Commun 2011;414:304–8.
72. Jang HS, Park KN, Kang CD, et al. Optical fiber SPR biosensor with sandwich assay for the detection of prostate specific antigen. Optics Comm 2009;282:2827–30.
73. Cao C, Kim JP, Kim BW, et al. A strategy for sensitivity and specificity enhancements in prostate specific antigen-1-antichymotrypsin detection based on surface plasmon resonance. Biosens Bioelectron 2006;21:2106–13.
74. Suwansa-ard S, Kanatharana P, Asawatreratanakul P, et al. Comparison of surface plasmon resonance and capacitive immunosensors for cancer antigen 125 detection in human serum samples. Biosens Bioelectron 2009;24:3436–41.

75. Mine N, Yamamoto S, Saito N, et al. CBP501-calmodulin binding contributes to sensitizing tumor cells to CDDP and BLM. Mol Cancer Therapy 2011;10:1929–38.

76. Ma J, Xin X, Meng L, et al. The marine-derived oligosaccharide sulfate (MdOS), a novel multiple tyrosine kinase inhibitor, combats tumor angiogenesis both in vitro and in vivo. PLoS One 2008;3:e3774.

77. Ahad AM, Zuohe S, Du-Cuny L, et al. Development of sulfonamide AKT PH domain inhibitors. Bioorg Med Chem 2011;19:2046–54.

78. Vicari D, Foy KC, Liotta EM, et al. Engineered conformation-dependent VEGF peptide mimics are effective in inhibiting VEGF signaling pathways. J Biol Chem 2011;286: 13612–25.

79. Matthews SB, Vielhauer GA, Manthe CA, et al. Characterization of a novel novobiocin analogue as a putative C-terminal inhibitor of heat shock protein 90 in prostate cancer cells. Prostate 2010;70:27–36.

80. Chang HH, Song Z, Wisner L, et al. Identification of a novel class of anti-inflammatory compounds with anti-tumor activity in colorectal and lung cancers. Invest New Drugs 2011. [Epub ahead of print].

81. Chen L, Pernazza D, Scott LM, et al. Inhibition of cellular Shp2 activity by a methyl ester analog of SPI-112. Biochem Pharmacol 2010;80:801–10.

82. Chen CH, Kuo SC, Huang LJ, et al. Affinity of synthetic peptide fragments of MyoD for Id1 protein and their biological effects in several cancer cells. J Pept Sci 2010;16: 231–41.

83. Liu Y, Pan Y, Xu Y. Binding Investigation of Integrin $\alpha_v\beta_3$ with its inhibitors by SPR technology and molecular docking simulation. J Biomol Screen 2010;15:131–7.

84. Qiu J, Xiao J, Han C, et al. Potentiation of tumor necrosis factor-$\alpha$-induced tumor cell apoptosis by a small molecule inhibitor for anti-apoptotic protein hPEBP4. J Biol Chem 2010;285:12241–7.

85. Erkizan HV, Scher LJ, Gamble SE, et al. Novel peptide binds EWS-FLI1 and reduces the oncogenic potential in Ewing tumors. Cell Cycle 2011;10:3397–408.

86. Bulut G, Hong SH, Chen K, et al. Small molecule inhibitors of ezrin inhibit the invasive phenotype of osteosarcoma cells. Oncogene 2011. [Epub ahead of print].

# Phosphorylcholine Self-Assembled Monolayer-Coated Quantum Dots: Real-Time Imaging of Live Animals by Cell Surface Mimetic Glyco-Nanoparticles

Shin-Ichiro Nishimura, PhD

**KEYWORDS**

- Phosphorylcholine thiol derivative
- Aminooxy-terminated thiol derivative • Quantum dots
- Sialyl-Lewis X antigen • Living animal imaging
- Tissue-specific targeting

Glycans are expected to be one of the potential signal molecules for controlling drug targeting/delivery or long-term circulation of biopharmaceuticals. However, the effect of the carbohydrates of artificially glycosylated derivatives on in vivo dynamic distribution profiles after intravenous injection of model animals remains unexplored because of the lack of standardized methodology and suitable platform. Recently, we established an efficient and versatile method for the preparation of multifunctional quantum dots (QDs) displaying common synthetic glycosides with excellent solubility and long-term stability in aqueous solution without loss of quantum yields. Combined use of an aminooxy-terminated thiol derivative, 11,11'-dithio bis[undec-11-yl 12-(aminooxyacetyl)amino hexa(ethyleneglycol)], and a phosphorylcholine derivative, 11-mercaptoundecylphosphorylcholine, provided QDs with novel functions for the chemical ligation of ketone-functionalized compounds and the prevention of nonspecific protein adsorption concurrently. In vivo near-infrared (NIR) fluorescence imaging of various carbohydrates after administration into the tail vein of the mouse found that distinct long-term delocalization over 2 hours can be achieved in cases of QDs modified with $\alpha$-sialic acid residue (Neu5Ac-PCSAM-QDs) and control multifunctional

Field of Drug Discovery Research, Graduate School of Life Science, Hokkaido University and Medicinal Chemistry Pharmaceuticals LLC, Sapporo 001-0021, Japan
*E-mail address:* shin@sci.hokudai.ac.jp

Clin Lab Med 32 (2012) 73–87
doi:10.1016/j.cll.2011.12.002
0272-2712/12/$ – see front matter © 2012 Elsevier Inc. All rights reserved.

quantum dots (PCSAM-QDs) while QDs bearing other common sugars such as $\alpha$-glucose (Glc-PCSAM-QDs), $\alpha$-mannose (Man-PCSAM-QDs), $\alpha$-fucose (Fuc-PCSAM-QDs), lactose (Lac-PCSAM-QDs), $\beta$-glucuronic acid (GlcA-PCSAM-QDs), $N$-acetyl-$\beta$-D-glucosamine (GlcNAc-PCSAM-QDs), and $N$-acetyl-$\beta$-D-galactosamine (GalNAc-PCSAM-QDs) residues accumulated rapidly (5–10 minutes) in the liver. Sequential enzymatic modifications of GlcNAc-PCSAM-QDs gave Gal$\beta$1,4GlcNAc-PCSAM-QDs (LacNAc-PCSAM-QDs), Gal$\beta$1,4(Fuc$\alpha$1,3)GlcNAc-PCSAM-QDs (Le$^x$-PCSAM-QDs), Neu5Ac$\alpha$2,3Gal$\beta$1,4GlcNAc-PCSAM-QDs (sialyl LacNAc-PC-SAM-QDs), and Neu5Ac$\alpha$2,3Gal$\beta$1,4(Fuc$\alpha$1,3)GlcNAc-PCSAM-QDs (sialyl Le$^x$-PC-SAM-QDs) in quantitative yield as monitored by direct Matrix Assisted Laser Desorption Ionization Time-of-flight Mass Spectrometry (MALDI-TOFMS) analyses. Live animal imaging uncovered for the first time that Le$^x$-PCSAM-QDs also distributed rapidly in the liver after intravenous injection and almost quenched over 1 hour in similar profiles to those of LacNAc-PCSAM-QDs and Lac-PCSAM-QDs. On the other hand, sialyl LacNAc-PCSAM-QDs and sialyl Le$^x$-PCSAM-QDs were still retained stably in whole body after 2 hours, while they showed significantly different in vivo dynamics in the tissue distribution, suggesting that structure/sequence of the neighboring sugar residues in the individual sialyl oligosaccharides might influence the final organ-specific distribution. These results clearly show the evidence of an essential role of the terminal sialic acid residue(s) for achieving prolonged in vivo lifetime and biodistribution of various glyco-PCSAM-QDs as a novel class of functional platforms for nanoparticles-based drug targeting/delivery. A standardized protocol using multifunctional PCSAM-QDs should facilitate live cell/animal imaging of ligand-displayed QDs using versatile NIR fluorescence photometry without influence of size-dependent accumulation/excretion pathway for nanoparticles (eg, viruses) greater than 10 nm in hydrodynamic diameter by the liver.

Although carbohydrates have been long thought as high potential ligands for targeting tissues and cells in the discovery research for drug delivery systems and novel biomarkers because of specific interaction with their cell surface receptors, the method that can illuminate endogenous lectins to be beneficial for this approach remains to be unexplored. Our attention is now directed toward the influence of scaffold materials carrying carbohydrates to the in vivo dynamics and organ-specific accumulation of the attached glycans. It should be noted that evaluating the effect of carbohydrate moiety of various natural/nonnatural glycoconjugates on biodistribution and its lifetime appears to be difficult independently from the influence by the structure/property of aglycone (nonglycan) moieties, notably, artificial scaffold materials and hydrophobic photosensitive probes as well as protein core structures in native glycoproteins. It is well known that glycans usually exhibit relatively weak affinity with their partner molecules, such as enzymes and cell surface receptors, even though specificity of the interaction may be very high.[1–4] To investigate the functional role of the carbohydrate itself for controlling glycoprotein circulation and distribution in vivo, it seems likely that advent of a novel class of simple glycoprotein model, in which aglycone-scaffold should entail general globular proteinlike structure/property and the potential to prevent nonspecific interaction with other biomolecules, cells, tissues, or artificial materials surfaces.

Gold nanoparticles carrying carbohydrates are one of the simplest and most versatile glycoprotein models for probing and investigating functional roles of glycans in vitro using atomic force microscopy, transmission electron microscopy (TEM), or surface plasmon resonance.[5–7] Because it has been documented by in vivo imaging that gold nanoparticles exhibit higher adsorption than iodine as x-ray contrast agent with less bone and tissue interference achieving better contrast with lower x-ray dose,[8] noninvasive imaging of the biodistribution of glycan-conjugated gold nanoparticles may become possible in the near future. However, quantum dots (QDs) are fluorescence semiconductor nanoparticles that have unique optical properties, including narrow band and size-dependent luminescence with broad absorption, long-term photo stability, and resistance to photobleaching.[9–12] An attractive application of QDs is the living cells/animals imaging by simple fluorescent measurements,[13–24] which is possible because of surface modifications with various biomolecules such as DNA,[25,26] peptides,[27,28] proteins,[29–31] antibodies,[32,33] and carbohydrates.[34–39] As a scaffold to display carbohydrates and investigate their functions, advantages of QDs are summarized as follows: (1) QDs can be detected and monitored in vivo by simple fluorescent photometric analysis without any special and expensive equipment. (2) Multiple carbohydrates can be displayed on a single QD, and the carbohydrate density on the single QD can be readily controlled. Thus, enhanced affinity with target molecules is expected as a result of the glycoside cluster effect.[1–4] (3) The QDs range in size between several nanometers and dozens of nanometers, the same level as typical folded proteins (~10 nm in diameter), and are suitable for designing a new class of glycoprotein models. It is, therefore, expected that the QDs will exhibit behavior and dynamics similar to those of common globular proteins distributing in living cells and animals. Because inorganic, metal-containing QDs are synthesized in organic solvents by coating with hydrophobic ligands, such as trioctylphosphine oxide (TOPO), it is obvious that surface modification of QDs is needed to improve solubility and stability in common physiologic conditions. Thus far, many water-soluble QDs have been developed by coating with a variety of thiols and copolymers based on poly(ethylene glycols) (PEG)-like structures. However, it is noteworthy that nanoparticle hydrodynamic diameter is a crucial design parameter in the development of potential diagnostic and therapeutic agents. In fact, QDs greater than 10 nm in hydrodynamic diameter were proved to be accumulated by the liver designed specifically to capture and eliminate nanoparticles, whereas smaller QDs less than 5.5 nm resulted in rapid renal excretion. Currently, there is no versatile QD platform mimicking typical folded proteins (~10 nm in diameter) to have satisfactory functions both for displaying glycans and reducing nonspecific interactions with abundant serum and cellular proteins without loss of quantum yield of the original QDs.

## QDS COATED BY PHOSPHORYLCHOLINE SELF ASSEMBLED MONOLAYERS AND AMINOOXY-FUNCTIONALIZED MONOTHIOL DERIVATIVE

We thought that the use of phospholipidlike derivatives was a potential alternative to PEGylation because phosphatidylcholine is the most abundant and indispensable lipid component of stable biomembrane. We hypothesized that combined use of a simple monothiol, 11-mercaptoundecylphosphorylcholine (PC-SH),[40–43] and an aminooxy-terminated thiol derivative, 11,11'-dithio bis[undec-11-yl 12-(aminooxyacetyl)amino hexa(ethyleneglycol)] (ao-SH),[44] should provide QDs with promising characteristics, such as much higher solubility, stability, and ability to display multiple ligands as well as biomembrane-mimetic surface properties. As shown in **Fig. 1**A, ao-SH was first used for the enrichment analysis of glycosphingolipids on gold nanoparticles as scaffold, namely glycosphingolipidomics,[44] and allowed for high throughput characterization of glycosphingolipids in terms of structural analysis and binding assay based on high sensitive surface plasmon resonance. It is well documented that aminooxy-functional groups as well as hydrazide groups displayed on such solid materials are nice tools that accelerate high throughput and quantitative glycomics.[45–47] In addition, our previous study found that simple glycans and

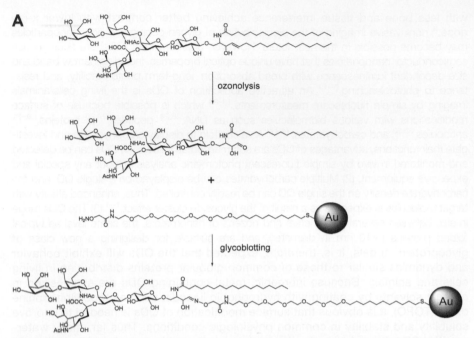

**Fig. 1.** Concepts and strategy for the preparation of glycosylated PCSAM-QDs. (*A*) "Glycob-lotting" is a chemical ligation-based enrichment of reactive ketones/aldehydes by particles having aminooxy/hydrazide functional groups. The scheme indicates an example of gold nanoparticles developed for a protocol of glycosphingolipidomics.[44] (*B*) Nonfouling surface coated by phosphorylcholine self-assembled monolayer. Glycosyltransferases can be immobilized in a highly oriented manner on PCSAM-Ag-magnetic beads.[43]

glycosphingolipid derivatives enriched by glycoblotting reaction with ao-SH on gold nanoparticles can be directly ionized from gold surfaces under general MALDI condition.[44–47] However, we found that phosphorylcholine self-assembled monolayers (SAMs) on silver-coated magnetic beads[43] can be applied for stable supporting materials to immobilize reusable engineered glycosyltransferases (see **Fig. 1**B), as this PCSAM becomes the suited platform for the specific interaction with *C*-terminal cationic amphiphilic peptide tag without any nonspecific protein adsorption. Taking these characteristics of 2 unique monothiol derivatives into account, this protocol seems to be advantageous for the construction of a variety of compound libraries displayed on the QD surfaces in a controlled density because the structure (quality) and quantity of molecules displayed on QDs might be determined concurrently by direct MALDI-TOF mass spectrometry without any purification or pretreatment procedure.

## PCSAM-QDS AS AN IDEAL SCAFFOLD FOR MOLECULAR DISPLAY

To assess the feasibility of PC-SH as a novel coating material for improving the properties of QDs surface, various PC-QDs were prepared by the simple ligand exchange reaction of PC-SH with TOPO-coated QDs (**Fig. 2**).[48] Reaction of PC-SH with commercially available TOPO-coated QDs with diameters in a range from 5.8 to 9.3 nm (CdSe/ZnS, $\lambda_{em}$ = 545, 565, 585, 605, and 655 nm) and synthetic TOPO-coated QDs of 11.7 nm (CdSeTe/CdS, $\lambda_{em}$ = 800 nm)[49–51] proceeded

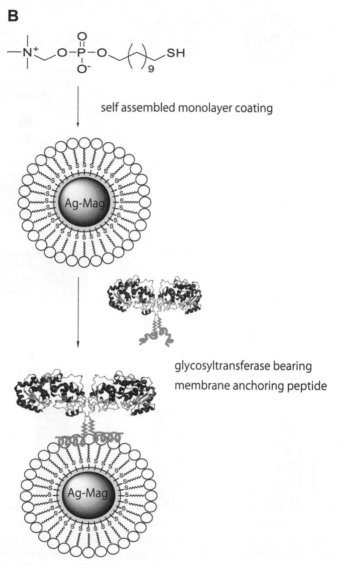

**Fig. 1** (*continued*).

smoothly and gave PC-QDs excellent solubility toward water. The surface modification with PC-SH was directly confirmed by MALDI-TOFMS, where the peaks at *m/z* 370.0 and 737.3 are simply assigned as PC-SH and disulfide form (PC-S-S-PC). Solubility toward water and the fluorescence intensity of PCSAM-QDs were evaluated by fluorescence correlation spectroscopy (FCS)[49–53] compared with those of simple PEG-QDs.[48] The fluorescence fluctuation of PCSAM-QDs was proved to be rapid and an ideal profile in the fitting curves with a single-component diffusion model, showing that PCSAM-QDs are well dispersed in water, whereas the results of PEG-QDs showed evidence of the formation of serious aggregation shortly after PEGylation of QDs surface. The diffusion

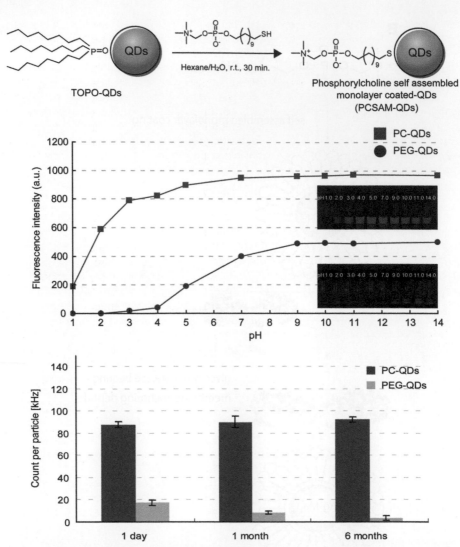

**Fig. 2.** Preparation and characterization of PCSAM-QDs. General protocol of the ligand exchange reaction from TOPO-QDs to PCSAM-QDs (*top*). The fluorescence intensity measured by spectrophotometer and photograph under ultraviolet irradiation at 365 nm of PCSAM-QDs and PEG-QDs in aqueous buffer solutions of various pH (*middle*). Fluorescence intensity per molecule was measured and estimated by FCS for the solutions of PCSAM-QDs and PEG-QDs stored in water at 4°C in the dark for 6 months (*bottom*).

coefficient and hydrodynamic diameter of PCSAM-QDs prepared from SeTe/CdS-type QDs were estimated to be 18.2 $\mu m^2 s^{-1}$ and 11.7 $\pm$ 1.5 nm based on the value of diffusion coefficient using 20 nm when fluospheres fluorescent beads (D = 10.4 $\mu m^2 s^{-1}$) was used as a standard material. On the contrary, PEG-QDs did not show any satisfactory fitting profile with either 1- or 2-component diffusion model, suggesting the importance of amphoteric nature of the PCSAM-QDs for preventing aggregation of QDs capped with monothiol derivatives.

Merit of the use of PC-SH is evident because PCSAM-QDs showed prominently long-term stability in water at 4°C and excellent resistance to an extensive range of pH (pH 2–14) compared with those of PEG-QDs (see **Fig. 2**). Surprisingly, PCSAM-QDs were stable for at least 6 months and the loss of fluorescence intensity was only 20% even at pH 3. This result suggests clearly that a balanced charge of zwitterions and minimized dipole of monothiol PC-SH are essential for the strong resistance of phosphorylcholine SAMs formed on QDs to aggregation because of their strong hydration capacity through electrostatic interaction. Moreover, it was also shown that monothiol anchor can stabilize QDs surface efficiently when such suitable amphoteric nature was incorporated into the hydrophilic head as well as good molecular packing of the hydrophobic linker moiety.

## GLYCO-PCSAM-QDS AS IDEAL GLYCOPROTEIN MODELS

General glycans released from naturally occurring glycoconjugates such as N-, O-glycans of glycoproteins and glycosphingolipid derivatives with oligosaccharide head groups can be directly captured by "glycoblotting,"[45–47] a promising method for chemoselective ligation of any reducing sugars or compounds bearing aldehyde/ketone by use of the aminooxy/hydrazide-functionalized materials. To display general carbohydrates and synthetic glycosides efficiently on the surface of QDs in combination with phosphorylcholine SAMs, it was considered that an aminooxy-functionalized ao-SH[44] containing 11-mercaptoundecyl moiety, an alkanethiol anchor group of PC-SH that allows an appropriate molecular packing structure of SAMs on QDs. To control the stereochemistry at an anomeric carbon of the reducing end of oligosaccharides even in cases of simple monosaccharides, we used versatile p-nitrophenyl glycosides as key starting materials. Various p-nitrophenyl glycosides readily prepared by conventional synthetic methods were converted into p-(4-oxopentanamido)-phenyl glycosides in high yields (**Fig. 3**). Reactions of glycosides with ao-PCSAM-QDs (ao-SH/PC-SH=2/8) proceeded smoothly in acetic acid buffer (pH 4.0) for 30 minutes at room temperature to afford glyco-PCSAM-QDs carrying β-Glc (Glc-PCSAM-QDs), α-Man (Man-PCSAM-QDs), α-Fuc (Fuc-PCSAM-QDs), β-GlcA (GlcA-PCSAM-QDs), β-GlcNAc (GlcNAc-PCSAM-QDs), β-GalNAc (GalNAc-PCSAM-QDs), β-Lac (Lac-PCSAM-QDs), and α-Neu5Ac (Neu5Ac-PCSAM-QDs), respectively. No unreacted aminooxy functional group ($H_2N-O-CH_2-$ at 4.17 ppm) was detected after glycoblotting, and the product generated by treating t with $I_2$ was also fully characterized by nuclear magnetic resonance (NMR) as the reasonable composition.[48] This clearly indicates that the ratio of glycan/PC on the QD surface can be controlled by that of ao-SH/PC-SH of the ao-PCSAM-QDs. TEM views showed that the diameters of ao-PCSAM-QDs and glyco-PCSAM-QDs were proved to be in a range from 7 nm (short side) to 10 nm (long side), and the results were in good agreement with those estimated by FCS (~11 nm).[48]

## GLYCO-PCSAM-QDS ARE VERSATILE TOOLS FOR REAL-TIME LIVE ANIMAL IMAGING

Glyco-PCSAM-QDs (CdSeTe/CdS) derived from NIR ao-PCSAM-QDs (**Fig. 3**) with excitation of 710 nm and emission of 800 nm were tested for live animal imaging to reduce nonspecific photoabsorption by biomolecules.[49–56] Initially, we assessed the real-time fluorescent monitoring of Lac-PCSAM-QDs and Neu5Ac-PCSAM-QDs in comparison with PCSAM-QDs as a control after injection into the vein of mouse tail (**Fig. 4**). It was reported that QDs of 5.5 nm or less drained from urine immediately and those of 5.5 nm or more accumulated in the liver, even though cysteine was used as a zwitterionic component in addition to DHLA,

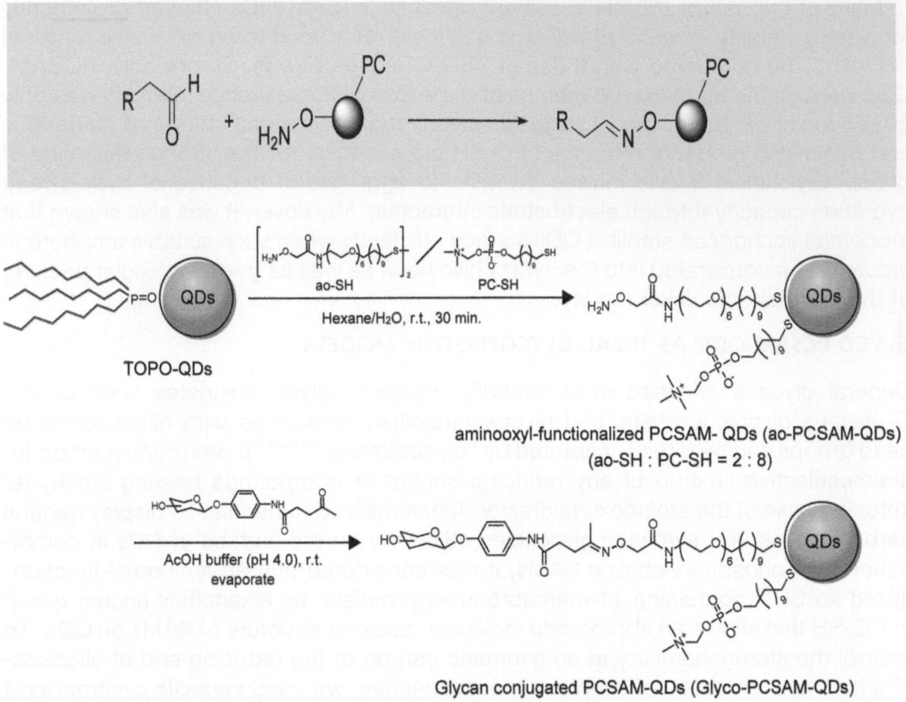

TOPO-QDs

ao-SH

PC-SH

Hexane/H₂O, r.t., 30 min.

aminooxyl-functionalized PCSAM- QDs (ao-PCSAM-QDs)
(ao-SH : PC-SH = 2 : 8)

AcOH buffer (pH 4.0), r.t.
evaporate

Glycan conjugated PCSAM-QDs (Glyco-PCSAM-QDs)

**Fig. 3.** A general protocol for the preparation of glyco-PCSAM-QDs by glycoblotting reaction with reactive ketones/aldehydes using ao-PCSAM-QDs.

cysteamine, and DHLA-PEG. Therefore, it seemed that PCSAM-QDs may distribute in the liver according to this size effect of QDs, because NIR PCSAM-QDs with 11.7 nm of diameter was tested for the current live animal imaging. It was also considered that Lac-PCSAM-QDs should accumulate in the liver shortly because of the hepatic asialoglycoprotein receptor[57–62] responsible for the specific interaction with terminal β-Galactosides of various oligosaccharides, while Neu5Ac-PCSAM-QDs might show a different organ distribution profile because of the effect of sialic acids. As anticipated, it was found that QDs bearing lactose began to accumulate in the liver immediately after administration. However, PCSAM-QDs and Neu5Ac-PCSAM-QDs did not distribute in any specific organ, indicating that nonfouling behavior observed in PCSAM-QDs is caused by the different mechanism from the resistance to nonspecific protein adsorption by QDs displaying cysteine having amino and carboxyl groups. Highly packing structure of monothiol phosphorylcholine-SAMs may provide QDs surface with specific nonfouling nature by strong hydration capacity through electrostatic interaction. This characteristic of PCSAM-QDs was not influenced by modification with Neu5Ac residues, whereas lactose moiety in Lac-PCSAM-QDs drastically altered PCSAM-QDs as liver-directed QDs. Interestingly, a photograph taken 10 minutes after the injection of other glyco-PCSAM-QDs showed that PCSAM-QDs having Glc, Man, Fuc, GlcNAc, and GalNAc also accumulated immediately in the liver and GlcA-PCSAM-QDs did not.[48] Surgery confirmed that the entire liver strongly fluoresced with Glc-PCSAM-QDs and GlcNAc-PCSAM-QDs and the bottom edge of the liver weakly fluoresced with GlcA-PCSAM-QDs (data not shown). These results clearly

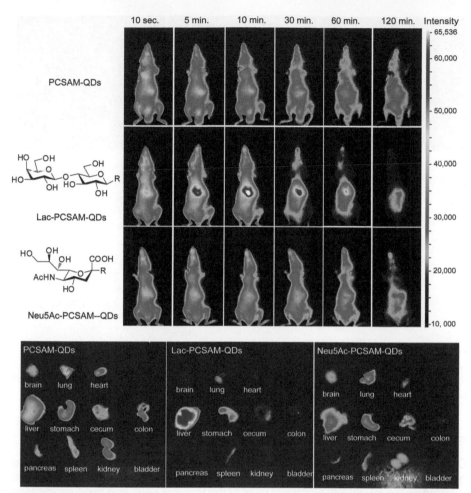

**Fig. 4.** Live animal imaging of glyco-PCSAM-QDs. Imaging of PCSAM-QDs, Lac-PCSAM-QDs, and Neu5Ac-PCSAM-QDs after injection of 100 pmole glyco-PCSAM-QDs (*top*). The mice were imaged using Lumazone equipped with Photometrics Cascade II EM CCD camera. QDs were excited with 710 nm, and emission filter was 800/12 nm bandpass filter. Photographs of major organs isolated from 3 tested mice (PCSAM-QDs, Lac-PCSAM-QDs, and Nue5Ac-PCSAM-QDs) 2 hours after administration (*bottom*).

showed that distinct long-term delocalization over 2 hours is observed only in cases of QDs modified with $\alpha$-sialic acid (Neu5Ac-PCSAM-QDs) and control PCSAM-QDs, whereas QDs bearing other popular neutral sugars were accumulated rapidly (5–10 minutes) in the liver. This trend was preliminarily demonstrated by photographs of fluoresced organs isolated from tested mice injected by 3 typical materials, PCSAM-QDs, Lac-PCSAM-QDs, and Neu5Ac-PCSAM-QDs (see **Fig. 4**). As shown in **Fig. 5**, confocal laser scanning microscope and TEM views of the liver tissue section derived from the mice injected by Lac-PCSAM-QDs suggested that QDs appeared to be incorporated into Kupffer cells and locate dominantly in endosomes, although mechanism of the intracellular trafficking of this class of nanoparticles remains to be unclear.

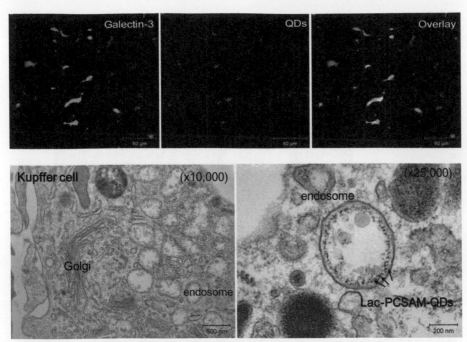

Fig. 5. Tissue imaging of Lac-PCSAM-QDs 2 hours after administration. Confocal laser scanning microscopic analysis suggested that Lac-PCSAM-QDs seem to locate mainly in the Kupffer cells expressing galectin-3 (*top*). TEM views indicated the intracellular distribution of Lac-PCSAM-QDs in the endosomes.

## GLYCOFORM-DEPENDENT TARGETING OF PCSAM-QDS

Considering that PCSAM-QDs were proved to be an ideal scaffold material mimicking general globular proteins with specific nonfouling surface, our interest was next focused on the insight into functional roles of the terminal sialic acid residues involved in the characteristic oligosaccharide moieties such as sialyl Lewis antigens. These antigens are known as an important core structures for possible ligands of mammalian lectins, such as selectins.[63–66] We have reported that simple sugar residues displayed on the surface of gold nanoparticles (3–8 nm in diameter) as well as synthetic dendrimers[67] can be further modified by some glycosyltransferases in the presence of sugar nucleotides. Conversion of a simple GlcNAc-PCSAM-QDs into more complicated glyco-PCSAM-QDs bearing LacNAc, Le$^x$, sialyl LacNAc, and sialyl Le$^x$ was performed successfully by treating sequentially with recombinant $\beta$1,4GalT, $\alpha$1,3FucT, and $\alpha$2,3Neu5Ac in the presence of suited sugar nucleotides under a general condition of enzymatic synthesis (**Fig. 6**).[67] As expected, all reactions proceeded smoothly and afforded target derivatives in quantitative yields, respectively, as monitored by MALDI-TOFMS.[48] Given the fact that globular proteinlike dendrimers with spherical molecular shape and size (~10 nm in diameter) are ideal polymer supports in the fully automated enzymatic glycan synthesis,[67] glyco-PCSAM-QDs appear to become a convenient glycoproteinlike model. These results clearly indicate that a strategy based on enzymatic sugar elongation of chemically synthesized simple glyco-PCSAM-QDs allows for the construction of highly complicated glycan-conjugated PCSAM-QDs library.

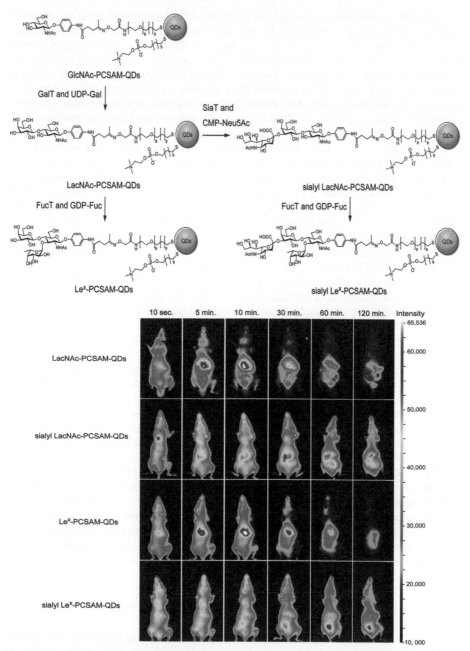

**Fig. 6.** Enzymatic synthesis of PCSAM-QDs bearing much more complicated carbohydrates from GlcNAc-PCSAM-QDs. Synthetic route of 4 glyco-PCSAM-QDs by means of 3 recombinant glycosyltransferases and sugar nucleotides (*top*). Live animal imaging of glyco-PCSAM-QDs carrying Lewis antigen-related oligosaccharides shows time course after injection of 100 pmole of these glyco-PCSAM-QDs.

In vivo NIR fluorescence imaging using PCSAM-QDs displaying LacNAc, Le$^x$, sialyl LacNAc, and sialyl Le$^x$ uncovered for the first time that Le$^x$-PCSAM-QDs are also accumulated rapidly (5~30 minutes) in the liver after intravenous injection and almost quenched over 1 hour in a similar profile to that of LacNAc-PCSAM-QDs (see **Fig. 6**). However, sialyl LacNAc-PCSAM-QDs and sialyl Le$^x$-PCSAM-QDs were still retained stably in the body after 2 hours while they exhibited significantly different in vivo dynamics in the tissue distribution observed by dissection at 2 hours after injection. It seemed that sialyl LacNAc-PCSAM-QDs appeared to locate spleen or intestine, and sialyl Le$^x$-PCSAM-QDs did not localize any organs, whereas Le$^x$-PCSAM-QDs distributed specifically in liver. These results suggest clearly that structure/sequence of the neighboring sugar residues in the individual sialylated oligosaccharides might influence significantly the organ-specific distribution after long-term circulation. Disappearance of fluorescence of these glyco-PCSAM-QDs after administration might be caused by the disintegration in the body without any leaking into urinary bladder or the urine. Metabolism and excretion pathway of PCSAM-QDs and individual sialic acid–containing glyco-PCSAM-QDs after injection into mice remain unclear, and there was no significant change in cell viability tested by using A549 cells between PCSAM-QDs and GlcNAc-PCSAM-QDs.[48]

We established a standardized procedure for the preparation of PCSAM-QDs, highly sensitive, stable, and nonfouling QDs coated by phosphorylcholine SAMs by means of a simple monothiol, 11-mercaptoundecylphosphorylcholine (PC-SH). Combined use with an aminooxy-terminated thiol derivative, 11,11'-dithio bis[undec-11-yl 12-(aminooxyacetyl)amino hexa(ethyleneglycol)] (ao-SH), allowed for the construction of an ideal glycoprotein model, namely, glyco-PCSAM-QDs, through the glycoblotting-based chemical ligation with ketone-functionalized synthetic glycosides. Further enzymatic modifications of simple glyco-PCSAM-QDs provided QDs having more complicated Lewis antigen-related oligosaccharides. It was found that nonfouling characteristic of highly stable PCSAM-QDs makes in vivo direct/real-time monitoring of glycan-specific interaction and distribution of glyco-PCSAM-QDs after injection into the vein of mouse tail possible. Live animal NIR fluorescence imaging of glyco-PCSAM-QDs showed the importance of the terminal sialic acid residues for achieving prolonged in vivo lifetime without size-dependent liver localization of nanoparticles. The advantage of this approach is clear because ao-PCSAM-QDs are novel classes of versatile scaffold for displaying a variety of compounds having reactive ketone/aldehyde as well as reducing sugars and synthetic glycosides used in this study. Considering the impact of current and emerging nanoparticle systems for the development of novel drug delivery and biomarkers, the current strategy would enable entirely novel classes of therapeutics.

## REFERENCES

1. Lee YC. Biochemistry of carbohydrate-protein interactions. FASEB J 1992;6:3193–200.
2. Lee YC, Lee RT. Carbohydrate-protein interactions: basis of glycobiology. Acc Chem Res 1995;28:321–7.
3. Mammen M, Choi SK, Whitesides GM. Polyvalent interactions in biological systems: implications for design and use of multivalent ligands and inhibitors. Angew Chem Int Ed 1998;37:2754–94.
4. Lundquist JJ, Toone EJ. The cluster glycoside effect. Chem Rev 2002;102:555–78.
5. de la Fuente JM, Eaton P, Barrientos AG, et al. Gold glyconanoparticles as water-soluble polyvalent models to study carbohydrate interactions. Angew Chem Int Ed 2001;40:2257–61.

6. Katz E, Willner I. Integrated nanoparticle-biomolecule hybrid systems: synthesis, properties, and applications. Angew Chem Int Ed 2004;43:6042–108.

7. Marradi M, Martin-Lomas M, Penades S. Glyconanoparticles polyvalent tools to study carbohydrate-based interactions. Adv Carbohydr Chem Biochem 2010;64:211–90.

8. Hainfeld JF, Slatkin DN, Focella TM, et al. Gold nanoparticles: a new X-ray contrast agent. Br J Radiol 2006;79:248–53.

9. Reed MA, Randall JN, Aggarwal RJ, et al. Observation of discrete electronic states in a zero-dimensional semiconductor nanostructure. Phys Rev Lett 1988;60:535–7.

10. Rossetti R, Nakahara S, Brus LE. Quantum size effects in the redox potentials, resonance Raman spectra, and electronic spectra of CdS crystallites in aqueous solution. J Chem Phys 1983;79:1086–8.

11. Gleiter H. Nanostructured materials. Adv Mater 1992;4:474–81.

12. Alivisatos AP. Semiconductor clusters, nanocrystals, and quantum dots. Science 1996;271:933–7.

13. Bruchez M Jr, Moronne M, Gin P, et al. Semiconductor nanocrystals as fluorescent biological labels. Science 1998;281:2013–16.

14. Chan WC, Nie S. Quantum dot bioconjugates for ultrasensitive nonisotopic detection. Science 1998;281:2016–18.

15. Jaiswal JK, Mattoussi H, Mauro JM, et al. Long-term multiple color imaging of live cells using quantum dot bioconjugates. Nat Biotechnol 2003;21:47–51.

16. Gao X, Cui Y, Levenson RM, et al. In vivo cancer targeting and imaging with semiconductor quantum dots. Nat Biotechnol 2004;22:969–76.

17. Medintz IL, Uyeda HT, Goldman ER, et al. Quantum dot bioconjugates for imaging, labelling and sensing. Nat Material 2005;4:435–46.

18. Uyeda HT, Medintz IL, Jaiswal JK, et al. Synthesis of compact multidentate ligands to prepare stable hydrophilic quantum dot fluorophores. Am Chem Soc 2005;127:3870–8.

19. Michalet X, Pinaud FF, Bentolila LA, et al. Quantum dots for live cells, in vivo imaging, and diagnostics. Science 2005;307:538–44.

20. Liu W, Choi HS, Zimmer JP, et al. Compact cysteine-coated CdSe(ZnCdS) quantum dots for in vivo applications. J Am Chem Soc 2007;129:14530–1.

21. Choi HS, Liu W, Misra P, et al. Compact cysteine-coated CdSe(ZnCdS) quantum dots for in vivo applications. Nat Biotechnol 2007;25:1165–70.

22. Liu W, Howarth M, Greytak AB, et al. Compact biocompatible quantum dots functionalized for cellular imaging. J Am Chem Soc 2008;130:1274–84.

23. Liu W, Greytak AB, Lee J, et al. Compact biocompatible quantum dots via RAFT-mediated synthesis of imidazole-based random copolymer ligand. J Am Chem Soc 2010;132:472–83.

24. Muro E, Pons Lequeux N, Fragola A, et al. Small and stable sulfobetaine zwitterionic quantum dots for functional live-cell imaging. J Am Chem Soc 2010;132:4556–7.

25. Dubertret B, Skourides P, Norris D, et al. In vivo imaging of quantum dots encapsulated in phospholipid micelles. Science 2002;298:1759–62.

26. Gill R, Willner I, Shweky I, et al. Fluorescence resonance energy transfer in CdSe/ZnS-DNA conjugates: probing hybridization and DNA cleavage. J Phys Chem B 2005;109:23715–19.

27. Cai W, Shin DW, Chen K, et al. Peptide-labeled near-infrared quantum dots for imaging tumor vasculature in living subjects. Nano Lett 2006;6:669–76.

28. Akerman M, Chan WC, Laakkonen P, et al. Nanocrystal targeting in vivo. Proc Natl Acad Sci 2002;99:12617–21.

29. Mattoussi H, Mauro JM, Goldman ER, et al. Self-assembly of CdSe-ZnS quantum dot bioconjugates using an engineered recombinant protein. J Am Chem Soc 2000;122: 12142–50.

30. Clapp AR, Medintz IL, Mauro JM, et al. Fluorescence resonance energy transfer between quantum dot donors and dye-labeled protein acceptors. J Am Chem Soc 2004;126:301–10.

31. Han H-S, Devaraj NK, Lee J, et al. Development of a bioorthogonal and highly efficient conjugation method for quantum dots using tetrazine-norbornene cycloaddition. Am Chem Soc 2010;132:7838–9.

32. Goldman ER, Balighian ED, Mattoussi H, et al. Avidin: a natural bridge for quantum dot-antibody conjugates. Am Chem Soc 2002;124:6378–82.

33. Wu X, Liu H, Liu J, et al. Immunofluorescent labeling of cancer marker Her2 and other cellular targets with semiconductor quantum dots. Nat Biotechnol 2003;21:41–6.

34. De la Fuente JM, Penades S. Glyco-quantum dots: a new luminescent system with multivalent carbohydrate display. Tetrahedron Asymm 2005;16:387–91.

35. Robinson A, Fang JM, Chou PT, et al. Probing lectin and sperm with carbohydrate-modified quantum dots. Chembiochem 2005;6:1899–1905.

36. Niikura K, Nishio T, Akita H, et al. Accumulation of O-GlcNAc-displaying CdTe quantum dots in cells in the presence of ATP. Chembiochem 2007;8:379–84.

37. Babu P, Sinha S, Surolia A, et al. Sugar-quantum dot conjugates for a selective and sensitive detection of lectins. Bioconj Chem 2007;18:146–51.

38. Niikura K, Nishio T, Akita H, et al. Oligosaccharide-mediated nuclear transport of nanoparticles. Chembiochem 2008;9:2623–7.

39. Yu M, Yang Y, Han R, et al. Polyvalent lactose-quantum dot conjugate for fluorescent labeling of live leukocytes. Langmuir 2010;26:8534–9.

40. Holmlin RE, Chen X, Chapman RG, et al. Zwitterionic SAMs that resist nonspecific adsorption of protein from aqueous buffer. Langmuir 2001;17:2841–50.

41. Tegoulia VA, Rao W, Kalambur AT, et al. Surface properties, fibrinogen adsorption, and cellular interactions of a novel phosphorylcholine-containing self-assembled monolayer on gold. Langmuir 2001;17:4396–404.

42. Chen S, Zheng J, Li L, et al. Strong resistance of phosphorylcholine self-assembled monolayers to protein adsorption: insights into nonfouling properties of zwitterionic materials. J Am Chem Soc 2005;127:14473–8.

43. Naruchi K, Nishimura S-I. Membrane-bound stable glycosyltransferases: highly oriented protein immobilization by a C-terminal cationic amphipathic peptide. Angew Chem Int Ed 2011;50:1328–31.

44. Nagahori N, Abe M, Nishimura S-I. Structural and functional glycosphingolipidomics by glycoblotting with an aminooxy-functionalized gold nanoparticle. Biochemistry 2009;48:583–94.

45. Nishimura S-I, Niikura K, Kurogochi M, et al. High-throughput protein glycomics: combined use of chemoselective glycoblotting and MALDI-TOF/TOF mass spectrometry. Angew Chem Int Ed 2004;44:91–6.

46. Nagahori N, Nishimura S-I. Direct and efficient monitoring of glycosyltransferase reactions on gold colloidal nanoparticles by using mass spectrometry. Chem Eur J 2006;12:6478–85.

47. Nishimura S-I. Toward automated glycan analysis. Adv Carbohydr Chem Biochem 2011;65:219–71.

48. Ohyanagi T, Nagahori N, Shimawaki K, et al. Importance of sialic acid residues illuminaterd by live animal imaging using phosphorylcholine self-assembled monolayers-coated quantum dots. J Am Chem Soc 2011;133:12507–17.

49. Bailey RE, Nie S. Alloyed semiconductor quantum dots: tuning the optical properties without changing the particle size. J Am Chem Soc 2003;125:7100–6.
50. Bailey RE, Strausburg JB, Nie SA. A new class of far-red and near-infrared biological labels based on alloyed semiconductor quantum dots. J Nanosci Nanotech 2004;4: 569–74.
51. Jin T, Fujii F, Komai Y, et al. Preparation and characterization of highly fluorescent, glutathione-coated near infrared quantum dots for in vivo fluorescence imaging. Int J Mol Sci 2008;9:2044–61.
52. Jin T, Fujii F, Sakata H, et al. Calixarene-coated water-soluble CdSe-ZnS semiconductor quantum dots that are highly fluorescent and stable in aqueous solution. Chem Commun 2005;2829-31.
53. Heuff RF, Swift JL, Cramb DT. Fluorescence correlation spectroscopy using quantum dots: advances, challenges and opportunities. Phys Chem Chem Phys 2007;9: 1870–80.
54. Frangioni JV. In vivo near-infrared fluorescence imaging. Curr Opin Chem Biol 2003;7:626–34.
55. Lim YT, Kim S, Nakayama A, et al. Selection of quantum dot wavelengths for biomedical assays and imaging. Mol Imaging 2003;2:50–64.
56. Choi HS, Ipe BI, Misra P, et al. Tissue- and organ-selective biodistribution of NIR fluorescent quantum dots. Nano Lett 2009;9:2354–9.
57. Lunney J, Ashwell G. A hepatic receptor of avian origin capable of binding specifically modified glycoproteins. Proc Natl Acad Sci U S A 1976;73:341–3.
58. Stockert RJ, Morell AG, Scheinberg H. The existence of a second route for the transfer of certain glycoproteins from the circulation into the liver. Biochem Biophys Res Commun 1976;68: 988–93.
59. Kawasaki T, Etoh R, Yamashina I. Isolation and characterization of a mannan-binding protein from rabbit liver. Biochem Biophys Res Commun 1978;81:1018–24.
60. Prieels J-P, Pizzo SV, Glasgow LR, et al. Hepatic receptor that specifically binds oligosaccharides containing fucosyl alpha1 leads to 3 N-acetylglucosamine linkages. Proc Natl Acad Sci U S A 1978;75:2215–19.
61. Baenziger J, Flete D. Galactose and N-acetylgalactosamine-specific endocytosis of glycopeptides by isolated rat hepatocytes. Cell 1980;22:611–20.
62. Ashwell G, Harford J. Carbohydrate-specific receptors of the liver. Ann Rev Biochem 1982;51:531–54.
63. Somers WS, Tang J, Shaaw GD, et al. Insights into the molecular basis of leukocyte tethering and rolling revealed by structures of P- and E-selectin bound to SLe(X) and PSGL-1. Cell 2000;103:467–479.
64. Varki A. Selectin ligands. Proc Natl Acad Sci U S A 1994;91:7390–7.
65. Rosen SD, Bertozzi CR. The selectins and their ligands. Curr Opin Cell Biol 1994;6: 663–73.
66. Rosen SD. Ligands for L-selectin: homing, inflammation, and beyond. Ann Rev Immunol 2004;22:129–56.
67. Matsushita T, Nagashima I, Fumoto M, et al. Artificial Golgi apparatus: globular protein-like dendrimer facilitates fully automated enzymatic glycan synthesis. Am Chem Soc 2010;132:16651–6.

# Gold Nanoparticle–Mediated Detection of Circulating Cancer Cells

Kiran Bhattacharyya, BS[a], Benjamin S. Goldschmidt, BS[a],
Mark Hannink, PhD[b,c], Stephen Alexander, PhD[d],
Aleksander Jurkevic, PhD[c], John A. Viator, PhD[d,c,e],*

**KEYWORDS**

- Antibody • Circulating tumor cells • EpCAM • Metastasis
- Optoacoustic

Circulating tumor cells (CTCs) are cells that undergo transitions that promote detachment from a solid tumor and allow them to travel in suspension through the blood and lymph systems to create secondary tumors. Detection of CTCs may allow earlier diagnosis, determine remission and relapse, and monitor response to therapy, as the concentration of CTCs has been shown to correlate with disease state.[1–3] We have been successful in detecting and capturing pigmented, circulating melanoma cells (CMCs) owing to their natural light-absorbing nature, though cancer cells of other types lack intrinsic color and cannot be detected without the addition of extrinsic optical absorbers. We investigated nonpigmented CTC detection using antibody-targeted gold nanoparticles in a breast cancer cell line, T47D (**Fig. 1**). The specific targeting of gold nanoparticles to breast cancer cells allowed us to repeat our earlier success with melanoma by detection of these cells in suspension in our photoacoustic flowmeter.

In addition to the direct clinical benefit of detecting CTCs, this system may be used to capture CTCs for clinically relevant cancer biology research. Malignant cancer cells

The authors acknowledge the support of the Department of Biological Engineering and the Christopher S. Bond Life Sciences Center at the University of Missouri. They acknowledge grant support from Missouri Life Sciences Research Board 09-1034 and NIH R21CA139186-0. The authors also thank the Life Sciences Undergraduate Research Opportunity Program at the University of Missouri, the University of Missouri Molecular Cytology Core, and the University of Missouri College of Engineering for financial support.

John A. Viator has invented photoacoustic flowmetry for in vitro detection of pathologic analytes in body fluids and has formed Viator Technologies Inc. to commercialize this technology.

[a] Department of Biological Engineering, University of Missouri, Columbia, MO 65212, USA
[b] Department of Biochemistry, University of Missouri, Columbia, MO 65212, USA
[c] Christopher S. Bond Life Sciences Center, University of Missouri, Columbia, MO 65211, USA
[d] Division of Biological Sciences, University of Missouri, Columbia, MO 65211, USA
[e] Department of Dermatology, University of Missouri, Columbia, MO 65211, USA
* Corresponding author. 240 Christopher Bond Life Sciences Center, Columbia, MO 65211-7310.
*E-mail address:* viatorj@missouri.edu

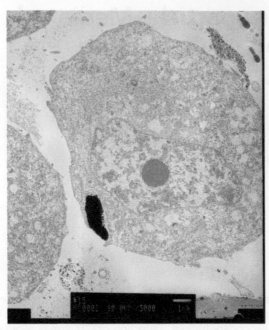

**Fig. 1.** A breast cancer cell with nanoparticles endocytosed into it.

have acquired not only genetic mutations that enable uncontrolled proliferation and tumor formation, but also the ability to leave the primary tumor and set up secondary tumor growths in other tissues throughout the body. Indeed, clinicians now appreciate that metastasis—the formation of multiple secondary tumors—is the primary cause of death in cancer patients. Multiple therapeutic options, including surgery, radiation, and chemotherapy, can be used to kill cancer cells in a primary tumor. Because of their singular importance in the pathogenesis of the disease, metastatic cancer cells represent the single most important therapeutic target for cancer treatment. A major goal of cancer research is to define the mechanisms that lead to metastasis and identify unique properties of metastatic cells that can be exploited for therapy.[4,5] Using photoacoustic flowmetry, it may be possible to capture CTCs and perform such studies to validate and enable future therapies.

Other methods are being investigated for detection of CTCs, including immuno-magnetic separation, polymerase chain reaction (PCR) methods, microfluidic capture, and conventional flow cytometry, though photoacoustic flowmetry allows sensitive detection and capture of intact CTCs in suspension.[6–15] This advantage allows further testing of the cells, including imaging or molecular and genetic assays. Conventional flow cytometry shares this advantage, but its implementation is not suited for detection of rare events, such as the case in CTCs in which only a few cells might be present among billions of normal blood cells in a 10-mL sample.

## BIOLOGY AND CLINICAL IMPORTANCE OF DETECTION OF CTCs

The detection and characterization of CTCs is a clinically important goal. For example, simply tracking the concentration of CTCs in the blood of patients over time will provide insight into the disease status of a patient and can be used to monitor the response of a patient to therapy. Further, information gained from molecular analyses of these CTCs can provide crucial information regarding the presence of specific DNA mutations or cell-surface proteins. Such molecular information can be of prognostic value in the clinic and can also provide new insights into fundamental questions of cancer biology.

A metastatic cell must leave the primary tumor and enter either the lymphatic system or the vasculature. Subsequently, the cell must invade distant tissue and proliferate to form a metastatic tumor.[16] Thus, metastatic cells are derived from cells that were, at one time, CTCs. However, the molecular characteristics of a CTC that enable it to seed sites of metastatic tumor growth are largely unknown.

A fundamental question is the relationship between CTCs and cancer stem cells (CSCs). CSCs, which are defined by their ability to form a tumor, are of considerable interest for both clinical assessments and for our understanding of cancer biology.[17] Although CSCs are thought to comprise a small percentage of cells in the primary tumor for many cancers, recent work has suggested that more than 25% of cells within a primary melanoma have the ability to form a tumor when transplanted into severely immunocompromised mice.[18]

Recent work with breast CSCs has suggested that the epithelial–mesenchymal transition (EMT) is a key determinant of the CSC phenotype.[19] Forced expression of transcription factors that regulate the EMT, including Twist1 and Snail, in mammary epithelial cells increases both tumorigenicity and expression of cell surface markers that are markers of breast CSCs.[19] Efforts have been made to identify the cell surface proteome of both tumor-derived cancer cells[20–24] and CTCs,[25,26] but expression of these proteins on cancer cells is very heterogeneous and the precise relationship of these markers to CSCs and tumorigenicity is not clear.[18,22] A promising candidate is CD271,[20] a marker for neural crest cells.

We propose that the EMT characteristics of a CTC will be a good predictor of its metastatic ability. The development of reliable assays that measure the EMT characteristics in CTCs could be used as prognostic clinical indicators of the likelihood that cancer patients will develop metastases. The characterization of CTCs, which relies on the ability to isolate human CTCs, will provide important biological information to make photoacoustic detection an important diagnostic tool.

## PHOTOACOUSTIC INTERACTIONS WITH NANOPARTICLES

The use of light as a diagnostic tool in biomedical engineering and research has grown considerably in recent years. Whereas most diagnostic procedures in biomedical optics exploit the optical nature of the light–tissue interaction, photoacoustics uses optical energy to generate an acoustic wave in tissue. The acoustic wave is a robust means for carrying information that is immune to the highly photon scattering and signal degrading nature of tissue. *Thus, photoacoustics combines the high selectivity of optical absorption of targeted cells and tissue with the strong signal-to-noise ratio inherent in ultrasound propagation, the ideal balance of optical and acoustic techniques.*

Our photoacoustic flowmeter introduces a new paradigm in CTC detection. In its present form, it targets pigmented cells directly and requires no molecular labeling (**Fig. 2**). Further, the system has the potential to be fully automated, requiring no human intervention. The system we propose to develop will perform enrichment and isolation as well as using a statistical classifier for detecting the presence of melanoma cells in the sample. The blood sample will be separated by two-phase flow principles, so that instead of continuous flow, microdroplets of cells suspended in

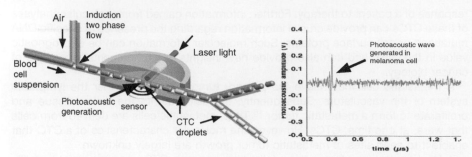

**Fig. 2.** The photoacoustic flowmeter separates continuous flow of blood cells with air bubbles. The resulting blood cell suspension droplets are irradiated by laser light. Droplets that contain CTCs generate photoacoustic waves that are sensed by an acoustic transducer. The waveform on the right shows a photoacoustic wave generated in a melanoma cell. These droplets are shunted off to a collection cuvette for further analysis. Negative bubbles are diverted for disposal.

saline separated by similar sized bubbles of air will pass through the detection area of the flow chamber. Droplets that generate photoacoustic waves will be directed to a holding cuvette that can be used for further analysis. Thus, not only can the presence and number of CTCs be determined, but also isolation of the CTC will allow verification of the test, along with the opportunity to conduct studies on CTCs to investigate questions about tumor biology and to provide clinically relevant information for management of advanced cancer.

Photoacoustics has been used to detect particles in suspension in a flowmetry scheme by Autrey and colleagues.[27] They performed measurements on latex microspheres and conducted analysis and modeling of the photoacoustic response with respect to shape and number. Detection of melanoma cells in suspension was first shown by Weight and colleagues.[28] We demonstrated the use of a photoacoustic flowmeter to detect melanoma cells with a limit of fewer than 10 CMCs at a time.

Further, in the article by Holan and coworkers,[29] we showed the efficacy of using the maximal overlap discrete wavelet transform (MODWT) to de-noise photoacoustic signals to improve detection of CMCs, in vitro.

Zharov and colleagues have developed a photoacoustic method in which CMCs are detected in vivo using a rabbit model.[30,31] This work is groundbreaking in that it is noninvasive. However, translating this detection to a human being may be problematic because the thicker tissue separating a detection device and blood vessels will cause optical and acoustic attenuation. Further, this method, because it is in vivo, precludes cell isolation and capture.

We have used photoacoustic principles and coupled them with flow cytometric concepts and created a photoacoustic flowmeter capable of detecting and enumerating small light-absorbing particles under flow. In contrast to conventional flow cytometry,[32,33] in which targeted cells are tagged to create fluorescent signals, we target cells with some pigment or light absorber to create high-frequency ultrasonic waves. In the photoacoustic flowmeter, the fluids are leukocytes suspended in phosphate-buffered saline (PBS) and air. Two-phase flow allows us to sequester any CTC in a localized volume so that capture and purification can be performed easily. In addition, the air barrier between droplets of PBS creates an acoustic free surface that limits photoacoustic signals to remain within its own droplet, thus preventing crosstalk from nearby droplets.[34,35]

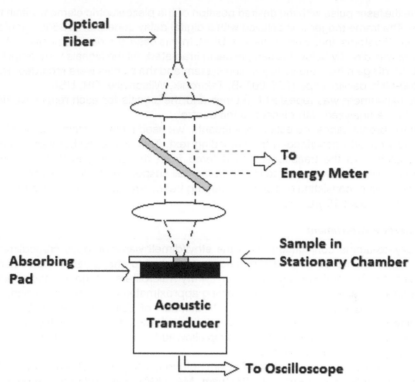

**Fig. 3.** The photoacoustic setup for measurements not under flow is shown here. This setup was used for the photoacoustic spectrum measurements. The flow measurements were performed in a similar manner, except that instead of a stationary chamber, the cell suspension was sent through the laser beam under flow through a cylindrical chamber.

## MATERIALS AND METHODS
### Photoacoustic Detection

The photoacoustic system used for this research consisted of a tunable Opotek Vibrant (Vibrant 355 II, Opotek, Carlsbad, CA, USA) 355 II Q-switched laser system to irradiate our samples pulsing at a wavelength of 532 nm. The laser pulsed at a 10-Hz repetition rate with approximate 5 ns duration. The average energy of the laser pulse at 532 nm was 3.5 mJ. The pulsed light beam was delivered to a glass microcuvette containing the sample of interest by use of an optical fiber. The microcuvette had a cylindrical hole ground in the center of the microscope slide with a diameter of 1.2 mm (**Fig. 3**). The microcuvette contained 5 $\mu$L of liquid sample and was coupled to an ultrasound transducer by ultrasound gel and an optical scattering pad. This scattering pad was made from acrylamide gel mixed with Intralipid (Abbot Laboratories, Chicago, IL, USA) to attenuate the laser beam and protect the transducer. The acoustic signal generated was then detected using the ultrasound transducer probe (RMV-708), attached to the Vevo 770 Imaging system (Visual Sonics Inc., Toronto, Ontatio, Canada) with 30 $\mu$m resolution and frame rates up to 240 frames per second (fps). The ultrasound imaging probe housed a single piezoelectric sensing element, which moved at the user-defined frame rate to collect lines of data within each frame. The ultrasound machine, set at 10 fps, was used to trigger the 10-Hz Q-switched laser to time the laser pulse with the desired position of the piezoelectric element within the probe. The frame trigger was delayed with a digital delay generator (DG535, Stanford Research Systems, Inc., Sunnyvale, CA, USA). In this case, the desired position of the element was directly below the sample being irradiated. All the signals were amplified with a 31-dB gain from the Vevo imaging system and the signals were recorded using the 200-MHz oscilloscope (TDS 2034B, Tektronix, Wilsonville, OR, USA).

The experiment was repeated five times and the signals for each respective time period were analyzed with respect to the control.

For the breast cancer detection experiments, we used a flow system instead of the stationary cuvette described in the preceding text. This flow chamber was acoustically matched to the transducer and differed from the cuvette in that a 1.5-mm cylindrical flow path was used to transport the cell suspension through a laser beam. The laser beam, consisting of a slowly diverging beam, irradiated a volume in the flow chamber of about 15 $\mu$L.

### Nanoparticle Attachment

Carboxyl-to-amine conjugation using the ethyl(dimethylaminopropyl) carbodiimide-N-Hydroxysuccinimide EDC-NHS procedure was used to attach carboxylated nanoparticles to the anti-EpCam antibody.[36] Fifty microliters of gold nanoparticles suspended in deionized (DI) water containing approximately $1.5 \times 10^{11}$ nanoparticles were incubated with 135 $\mu$L of a 0.3 $\mu$M solution of EDC dissolved in DI water combined with 200 $\mu$L of a 0.4 $\mu$M solution of NHS for 15 minutes at room temperature, approximately 22°C. This step allowed for the activation of the carboxyl bonds on the nanoparticle surface.

After 15 minutes, 2 $\mu$L of of anti-EpCam solution, 100 $\mu$g/mL (Thermo Scientific: Pierce Protein Research Products, Waltham, MA, USA), was added to the previous solution of now carboxyl-activated gold nanoparticles and allowed to react for 2 hours at room temperature.

After 2 hours, 613 $\mu$L of DI water was added to the previous solution to bring the total volume to 1 mL to make consequent calculations simpler. Next, 6.67 $\mu$L of the gold nanoparticle suspension was incubated with $1 \times 10^6$ T47D breast cancer cells suspended in 1 mL of PBS solution for 1 hour to allow the nanoparticles to attach to the cancer cell.

After 1 hour, the cell solution was cleaned of excess nanoparticles by centrifugation. This was repeated three times at 1400 rpm for 12 minutes and the cells were washed after each cycle. Cells with attached nanoparticles were imaged using a fluorescence microscope (LSM 510 META NLO, Carl Zeiss, Inc., Oberkochen, Germany).

### Rhodamine Attachment to Nanoparticles

To verify nanoparticle attachment to the breast cancer cells, we conjugated rhodamine dye molecules to the nanoparticles. Thus, fluorescence imaging could be used to verify nanoparticle attachment.

The same carboxyl-to-amine conjugation using the EDC-NHS procedure was used to attach rhodamine 6G, which has two carboxyl groups per molecule, to the anti-EpCam-AuNP conjugate, where AuNP refers to gold nanoparticle.

Eighty microliters of 1 $\mu$M rhodamine solution were dissolved in DI water and incubated with 135 $\mu$L of a 0.3 $\mu$M solution of EDC dissolved in DI water combined with 200 $\mu$L of a 0.4 $\mu$M solution of NHS for 15 minutes at room temperature, approximately 22°C. This step activated the carboxyl groups on the rhodamine molecules.

After 15 minutes, 585 $\mu$L of the anti-EpCam-AuNP conjugate prepared earlier was added to the rhodamine solution and allowed to react for 12 hours at 4°C to attach the

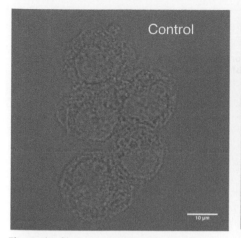
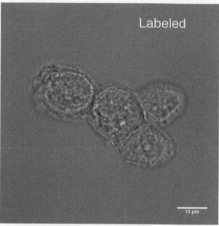

**Fig. 4.** (*Left*) Control T47D cells incubated in the presence of gold nanoparticles not conjugated to anti-EpCAM show no nanoparticle enhancement. (*Right*) T47D cells incubated with nanoparticles targeting anti-EpCAM show attachment by rhodamine fluorescence.

rhodamine to the antibody on the anti-EpCam-AuNP conjugate. After 12 hours, the excess unreacted rhodamine was cleaned out of the solution by centrifugation at 6000 rpm for 10 minutes. This was repeated three times. The high centrifugation speed was necessary to ensure that the rhodamine–antibody–AuNP conjugate would form a pellet.

Ten microliters of this new conjugate was incubated with $1 \times 10^6$ T47D cells in 1 mL of PBS for 1 hour. A different cell suspension with $1 \times 10^6$ T47D cells, in 1 mL as well, was first incubated with 2 $\mu$L of excess anti-EpCam stock solution to block EpCam receptors on the cell surface and then incubated with 10 $\mu$L of rhodamine–antibody–AuNP solution for 1 hour. Both cell suspensions were cleaned by centrifugation at 1400 rpm for 12 minutes. The cleaning process was repeated three times for both suspensions. The receptor blocked cells serve as the control to show the specificity of the AuNP target.

### Photoacoustic Spectrum of Nanoparticles

We performed spectroscopic analysis of the gold nanoparticles using a white light transmission spectrometer and compared it to the photoacoustic response as a function of wavelength from 480 to 570 nm. The spectrometer was an Ocean Optics HR200 (Ocean Optics, Dunedin, FL, USA) with a tungsten arc lamp source. To compare the photoacoustic response directly to the white light measurements, we normalized the absorbance by the highest measured value to obtain a relative absorbance for both spectra. The photoacoustic measurements were performed as described previously in the non-flowing setup. We used 4 $\mu$L of stock gold nanoparticle suspension and tested the photoacoustic response in 10-nm increments. The same sample was irradiated in the entire range of laser wavelengths.

### Photoacoustic Detection of Tagged Breast Cancer Cells

Using antibody targeted T47D breast cancer cells, we performed serial dilutions and tested them in the photoacoustic flowmeter. Because we were not capturing

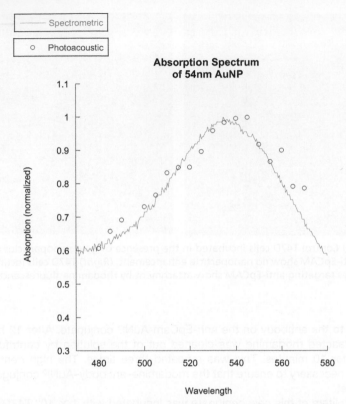

**Fig. 5.** The photoacoustic peak absorption closely matches that indicated by white light spectroscopy. The peaks, about 540 nm, are to the 532-nm wavelength we used. This wavelength was chosen because it is the second harmonic of an Nd:YAG laser.

cells, we used a continuous flow of cell suspension in these experiments. We used laser wavelength of 532 nm with 4.1 mJ of laser energy. The beam volume through the detection chamber was 15 $\mu$L and the flow rate was 100 $\mu$L/min. Each waveform was from a single laser pulse; thus no waveform averaging was performed.

## RESULTS
### Attachment of Nanoparticles to Breast Cancer Cells

**Fig. 4** shows selective attachment of gold nanoparticles to breast cancer cells, verified by fluorescence measurements. The control cells were exposed to fluorescently labeled gold nanoparticles while the others were exposed to gold nanoparticles conjugated to the EpCAM antibody. The figure shows no fluorescence on the control, whereas EpCAM-targeted cells show significant nanoparticle attachment.

### Photoacoustic Spectrum of Nanoparticles

**Fig. 5** shows the photoacoustic spectrum of the nanoparticles alongside the spectrum obtained from white light spectroscopy. The photoacoustic peak is approximately 540 nm, while the white light peak is at about 538 nm.

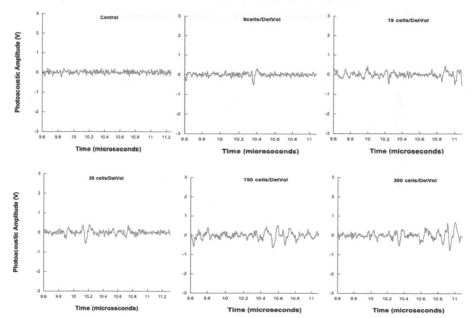

**Fig. 6.** These data show photoacoustic waves generated in tagged breast cancer cells. While the number of peaks do not correlate with expected cell number, the total photoacoustic energy, indicated by the area under the pressure waves, has an increasing trend with increasing cell concentration.

### Photoacoustic Detection of Tagged Breast Cancer Cells

Photoacoustic waveforms from irradiating 9, 19, 38, 150, and 300 tagged breast cancer cells are shown along with a control in **Fig. 6**. In each case, the number of photoacoustic waves is less than indicated by the expected number of cancer cells. However, total energy indicated by the area under the curve of each pressure wave shows an increasing trend.

**Fig. 7** shows the integrated pressure as a function of cell concentration. This figure approximates the total photoacoustic energy obtained and correlates it to the expected cell number.

### DISCUSSION

We have presented results showing successful nanoparticle attachment to the T47D breast cancer cell line. These nanoparticles provided optical contrast resulting in photoacoustic generation in our flowmeter. Although we did not specifically show single breast cancer cell detection, we claim that this system may be capable of such detection. Our results were confounded by cell clumping (**Fig. 8**). However, we believe that single cell detection is possible, and in the clinical case, CTC clumping would not necessarily be present.

Using a tunable laser system, we can target different absorption peaks, such as those associated with dyed microspheres or nanoparticles of different diameters. The photoacoustic response as a function of wavelength showed a peak close to 540 nm. Using the second harmonic of the Nd:YAG laser, we were successful in exploiting high optical absorption. In future applications, different absorption peaks can be targeted with the tunable ability of an optical parametric oscillator pumped laser system.

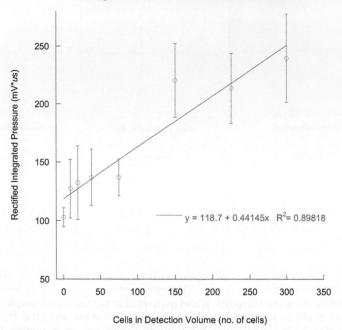

**Integrated Pressure vs. Cell Concentration**

$y = 118.7 + 0.44145x$   $R^2 = 0.89818$

Cells in Detection Volume (no. of cells)

**Fig. 7.** Integrated pressure provides a means to correlate with cell number in the detection volume. This measure, in contrast to numbers of photoacoustic waveforms, indicates breast cancer cells may be aggregating to form clusters of light absorbers.

## Justification of Single-Cell Detection

Single cells and clusters of cells cannot yet be differentiated by the photoacoustic flowmetry system. Therefore, relating photoacoustic events to the number of cells being irradiated in the flow chamber must take into account if the cell suspension being tested has groups of clustered cells along with single cells.

**Fig. 9** gives the probability, $P(c)$, that any given cell in the sample is in a cluster of size $c$. Any random cell has an approximately 29% chance of being in a cluster with 9 or more other cells. This distribution was arrived at by counting, with the aid light microscopy, 563 cells in the sample, some of which were found to be in these clusters and others were individually dispersed. Therefore, the total number of clusters and single cells in a cell suspension can be calculated if the total number of cells is known. For example, 9 cells/detection volume, when the detection volume is 15 $\mu L$, is 600 cells/mL. Given that the clustering distribution applies to this sample, there would be 195 clusters/mL, including single cells that have a cluster size of 1.This was arrived at with the following formula:

$N * P(c)/c$

Where N is the number of cells per milliliter, 600 in this case, and $P(c)$ and $c$ were previously defined.

This concentration of 195 clusters/mL relates better to the number of photoacoustic events expected in the detection volume than the total cell concentration of 600 cells/mL. The total number of photoacoustic events in 14 waveforms was counted and found to be 38, each waveform representing a signal from a 15-$\mu L$ volume, for a

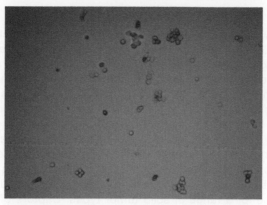

**Fig. 8.** Micrograph shows breast cancer cells clumping. Because of the close spatial relationship of clumped cells, a single photoacoustic waveform is generated, although it has commensurately greater energy.

total of 210 $\mu$L. The expected number of clusters in that volume calculated from the concentration would be (195) * (0:210) = 40:95, or approximately 41 clusters.

The agreement between the number of counted events, 38, and the expected number of clusters, 41, is an indication of robust detection. The disparity can be attributed to a random deviation from the expected value. According to the Poisson distribution, when the expected value is 41, there is a 6.2% chance of measuring exactly 41 events and a 5.7% chance of measuring exactly 38 events. Though the probabilities are different, a distinction between them can be made only with a very large sample size.

This is a strong indication that almost all, if not every cluster, including single cells that have a cluster size of 1 cell, were detected by the flowmetry system.

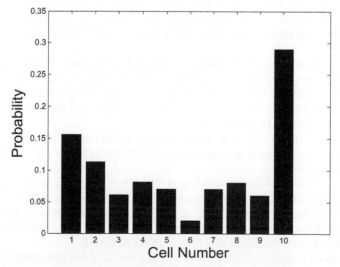

**Fig. 9.** Histogram showing probabilities of cells in each clump during the photoacoustic flow test.

## SUMMARY

Photoacoustic flowmetry has been used to detect pigmented particles in body fluids, most notably circulating melanoma cells in blood samples of metastatic melanoma patients. Exploiting the plasmon resonance of gold nanoparticles and the ability to specifically target cancer cell surface proteins, photoacoustic flowmetry may be used to detect nonpigmented CTCs. We targeted the EpCAM receptors to attach 50-nm gold nanoparticles to a breast cancer cell line, T47D. After determining the absorption peak and thus the most sensitive laser wavelength, we performed serial dilution trials to show detection of small numbers of breast cancer cells in suspension. Although some cell clumping may have altered some of our results for cell counting, it is feasible to use gold nanoparticles to detect and capture CTCs in a photoacoustic flowmeter. This ability may allow an earlier clinical diagnosis and management of metastatic disease for a range of solid tumor types. Capture of CTCs may also allow cell specific molecular analysis and a new paradigm for personalized cancer therapy.

## REFERENCES

1. Paterlini-Brechot P, Benali NL. Circulating tumor cells (CTC) detection: clinical impact and future directions. Cancer Lett 2007; 253:180–204.
2. Cristofanilli M, Braun S. Circulating tumor cells revisited. JAMA 2010;303:1092.
3. Gage T, Fan SL. What goes around, comes around: a review of circulating tumor cells analysis. 2010;11:18.
4. Bonnomet A, Brysse A, Tachsidis A, et al. Epithelial-to-mesenchymal transitions and circulating tumor cells. J Mammary Gland Biol Neoplasia 2010:1–13.
5. Maheswaran S, Haber DA. Circulating tumor cells: a window into cancer biology and metastasis. Curr Opin Genet Dev 2010;20(1):96–9.
6. Chang YC, Ye JY, Thomas TP, et al. Fiber-optic multiphoton flow cytometry in whole blood and in vivo. J Biomed Opt 2010;15:047004.
7. Okegawa T, Hayashi K, Hara H, et al. Immunomagnetic quantification of circulating tumor cells in patients with urothelial cancer. Int J Urol 2010;17:254–8.
8. Xu T, Lu B, Tai YC, et al. A cancer detection platform which measures telomerase activity from live circulating tumor cells captured on a microfilter. Cancer Res 2010; 70:6420.
9. Nagrath S, Sequist LV, Maheswaran S, et al. Isolation of rare circulating tumour cells in cancer patients by microchip technology. Nature 2007;450:1235–9.
10. Riethdorf S, Fritsche H, Muller V, et al. Detection of circulating tumor cells in peripheral blood of patients with metastatic breast cancer: a validation study of the CellSearch system. Clin Cancer Res 2007;13:920–8.
11. Zheng S, Lin H, Liu JQ, et al. Membrane microfilter device for selective capture, electrolysis and genomic analysis of human circulating tumor cells. J Chromatogr 2007;1162:154–61.
12. Zabaglo L, Ormerod MG, Parton M, et al. Cell filtration-laser scanning cytometry for the characterization of circulating breast cancer cells. Cytometry A 2003;55(2):102–8.
13. Gogas H, Kefala G, Bafaloukus D, et al. Prognostic significance of the sequential detection of circulating melanoma cells by RT-PCR in high-risk melanoma patients receiving adjuvant interferon. Br J Cancer 2003;88:981–2.
14. Pellegrino D, Bellina C, Manca G, et al. Detection of melanoma cells in peripheral blood and sentinel lymph nodes by RT-PCR analysis: a comparative study with immunochemistry. Tumori 2000;86:336–8.

15. Berking C, Schlupen EM, Schraeder A, et al. Tumor markers in peripheral blood of patients with malignant melanoma: multimarker RT-PCR versus a luminoimmunometric assay for S-100. Arch Dermatol Res 1999;291:479–84.
16. Gupta GP, Massague J. Cancer metastasis: building a framework. Cell 2006;127: 679–95.
17. Gupta PB, Chaffer CL, Weinberg RA. Cancer stem cells: mirage or reality? Nature Med 2009;15:1010–2.
18. Quintana E, Shackleton M, Sabel MS, et al. Efficient tumour formation by single human melanoma cells. Nature 2008;456:593–8.
19. Mani SA, Guo W, Liao MJ, et al. The epithelial-mesenchymal transition generates cells with properties of stem cells. Cell 2008;133:704–15.
20. Boiko AD, Razorenova OV, Rijn M, et al. Human melanoma-initiating cells express neural crest nerve growth factor receptor CD271. Nature 2010;466:133–7.
21. Cools-Lartigue JJ, McCauley CS, Marshall JCA, et al. Immunomagnetic isolation and in vitro expansion of human uveal melanoma cell lines. Mol Vis 2008;14:50.
22. Held MA, Curley DP, Dankort D, et al. Characterization of melanoma cells capable of propagating tumors from a single cell. Cancer Res 2010;70:388.
23. Kaufman KL, Belov L, Huang P, et al. An extended antibody microarray for surface profiling metastatic melanoma. J Immunol Methods 2010:23–34.
24. Petermann KB, Rozenberg GI, Zedek D, et al. CD200 is induced by ERK and is a potential therapeutic target in melanoma. J Clin Invest 2007;117:3922–9.
25. Kitago M, Koyanagi K, Nakamura T, et al. mRNA expression and BRAF mutation in circulating melanoma cells isolated from peripheral blood with high molecular weight melanoma-associated antigen-specific monoclonal antibody beads. Clin Chem 2009;55:757.
26. Nezos A, Lembessis P, Sourla A, et al. Molecular markers detecting circulating melanoma cells by reverse transcription polymerase chain reaction: methodological pitfalls and clinical relevance. Clin Chem Lab Med 2008;47:1–11.
27. Autrey T, Egerev S, Foster NS, et al. Counting particles by means of optoacoustics: potential limits in real solutions. Rev Sci Instrum 2003;74:628–31.
28. Weight RM, Dale PS, Caldwell CW, et al. Photoacoustic detection of metastatic melanoma cells in the human circulatory system. Opt Lett 2006:2998–3000.
29. Holan SH, Viator JA. Automated wavelet denoising of photoacoustic signals for circulating melanoma cell detection and burn image reconstruction. Phys Med Biol 2008;53:N227.
30. Zharov VP, Galanzha EI, Shashkov EV, et al. Photoacoustic flow cytometry: principle and application for real-time detection of circulating single nanoparticles, pathogens, and contrast dyes in vivo. J Biomed Opt 2007;12:051503.
31. Zharov VP, Galanzha EI, Shashkov EV, et al. In vivo photoacoustic flow cytometry for monitoring of circulating single cancer cells and contrast agents. Opt Lett 2006;31: 3623–5.
32. Laerum OD, Farsund T. Clinical application of flow cytometry: a review. Cytometry 1981;2:1–13.
33. Barlogie B, Raber MN, Schumann J, et al. Flow cytometry in clinical cancer research. Cancer Res 1983;43:3982.
34. Jensen F, Kuperman WA, Porter MB, et al. Computational ocean acoustics. Melville (NY): American Institute of Physics; 1995.
35. Blackstock DT. Fundamentals of physical acoustics. New York: Wiley-Interscience; 2001.
36. Grabarek Z, Gergely J. Zero-length crosslinking procedure with the use of active esters. Anal Biochem 1990;185:131–5.

# Index

*Note:* Page numbers of article titles are in **boldface** type.

### A

Activated leukocyte cell adhesion molecule, surface plasmon resonance for, 50, 52
Alpha-fetoprotein, surface plasmon resonance for, 53
Aminoxy-terminated thio derivatives, of phosphorylcholine, in quantum dots, **73–87**
Animal imaging, phosphorylcholine self-assembled monolayer-coated quantum dots for, **73–87**
Antibody arrays, for biomarkers, **33–45**
    description of, 35, 37
    examples of, 35
    labeling of, 36, 38–40
    panels for, 33–35, 37
    printing methods for, 36
    reproducibility of, 41–42
    sensitivity and specificity of, 40–41
    stability of, 42
    surface properties of, 35–36
Apoptosis
    dendrimers for, 15–16
    nanodots for, 19–20
Ataxia-telangiectasia-mutated kinase, surface plasmon resonance for, 66
Aurora kinases, surface plasmon resonance for, 63

### B

Bialys, nanoscale, 26–27
Bio-barcode assay, for prostate-specific antigen, 22
Biochips, nanoscale, for oral cancer biomarkers, 19
Biomarkers
    antibody arrays for, **33–45**
    for early detection, 22
    surface plasmon resonance for, **47–72**
Biomimetic nanoparticles, 25
Biosensors, nanoscale, 18
Bismuth sulfide, as contrast agent, for computed tomography, 23–24
Bladder cancer, antibody arrays for, 37
Bombesin, dendrimer nanoparticles with, 25
Breast cancer
    antibody arrays for, 37
    circulation tumor cell detection in, **89–101**
    photothermal therapy for, 27
    RNA quantification for, 2, 5
    surface plasmon resonance for, 52, 60
Bubbles, nanoscale, for ultrasound, 28–29

Clin Lab Med 32 (2012) 103–109
doi:10.1016/S0272-2712(12)00014-5
0272-2712/12/$ – see front matter © 2012 Elsevier Inc. All rights reserved.

# Moving?

## Make sure your subscription moves with you!

To notify us of your new address, find your **Clinics Account Number** (located on your mailing label above your name), and contact customer service at:

Email: journalscustomerservice-usa@elsevier.com

800-654-2452 (subscribers in the U.S. & Canada)
314-447-8871 (subscribers outside of the U.S. & Canada)

Fax number: 314-447-8029

**Elsevier Health Sciences Division**
**Subscription Customer Service**
**3251 Riverport Lane**
**Maryland Heights, MO 63043**

\*To ensure uninterrupted delivery of your subscription, please notify us at least 4 weeks in advance of move.

Printed and bound by CPI Group (UK) Ltd, Croydon, CR0 4YY
03/10/2024
01040454-0009